# Symptoms of Unknown Origin

*A Medical Odyssey*

# Symptoms of Unknown Origin

*A Medical Odyssey*

Clifton K. Meador, M.D.

Vanderbilt University Press
Nashville 2005

This book is printed on acid-free paper.
Manufactured in the United States of America

The prologue, "First Patient, 1952," was originally published in part in *Med School: A Collection of Stories, 1951 to 1955* (Nashville: Hillsboro Press, 2003). The patient in Chapter 1 was reported in abbreviated form in "The Person with the Disease," *Journal of the American Medical Association* 268 (1992):35. A modified report of Miss Cootsie, Chapter 3, appeared in "A Lament for Invalids," *Journal of the American Medical Association* 265 (1991):1374–75. A version of the story of Vance Vanders in Chapter 4 appeared in abbreviated form in "Hex Death: Voodoo Magic or Persuasion?" *Southern Medical Journal* 85 (1992):244–47.

Library of Congress Cataloging-in-Publication Data

Meador, Clifton K., 1931–
Symptoms of unknown origin : a medical odyssey / Clifton K. Meador.—
    1st ed. p. ; cm.
Includes bibliographical references and index.
ISBN 0-8265-1473-1 (cloth : alk. paper)
ISBN 0-8265-1474-X (pbk. : alk. paper)
    1. Clinical medicine—Case studies. 2. Diagnostic errors. 3. Medical
misconceptions. 4. Medicine—Philosophy. [DNLM: 1. Clinical Medicine—
Anecdotes. 2. Diagnostic Errors—Anecdotes. 3. Philosophy, Medical—
Anecdotes. 4. Physician-Patient Relations—Anecdotes. ]    I. Title.
RC66.M43 2005    616—dc22        2004028858

# Contents

Acknowledgments    vii

Introduction    ix

Prologue    1

1    An Unlikely Lesson from a Medical Desert    5

2    Texas Heat    15

3    Dr. Drayton Doherty and Miss Cootsie    20

4    All Some Patients Need Is Listening and Talking    27

5    Diagnoses Without Diseases    33

6    The Woman Who Believed She Was a Man    40

7    Mind and Body    49

8    Sweet Thing    55

9    New Clinical Interventions    61

10   Florence's Symptoms    66

11   Symptoms without Disease    81

12   Looking Back on Fairhope    95

13   The Diarrhea of Agnes    102

14   Dr. Jim's Breasts    108

15   The Woman Who Would Not Talk    114

16   The Woman Who Could Not Tell
     Her Husband Anything    124
17   Staying out of God's Way    133
18   A Paradoxical Approach    142
19   You Can't Be Everybody's Doctor    150
20   In Tune with the Patient    155

     Bibliography    165
     Index    169

# Acknowledgments

I appreciate all the help and encouragement I have received from my family, colleagues, and friends.

The following physicians reviewed earlier drafts of the book and made helpful suggestions and criticisms: Dean Steven Gabbe, Dean James Pittman, Dr. Jim Pichert, Dr. Kevin Soden, Dr. Taylor Wray, Dr. Eric Chazen, Dr. George Hansberry, Dr. John D. Thompson, Dr. Betty Ruth Speir, Dr. Kelley Avery, Dr. Eric Neilson, Dr. John Johnson, Dr. Norton Hadler, Dr. Ximena Paez, Dr. Julius Linn, Dr. Joseph Merrill, Dr. George Lundberg, Dr. Stephen Bergman, Dr. Abraham Verghese, Dr. John Newman, Dr. Albert Coker, and Dr. Caldwell DeBardeleben.

Colleagues and friends who helped me include Anita Smith, John Egerton, Fran Camacho, Cathy Taylor, Amy Minert, Joe Baker, Libbie Dayani, James Lawson, Stephen and Pamela Salisbury, Virginia Fuqua-Meadows, Lynn Fondren, Patty DeBardeleben, Diana Marver, Susanne Brinkley, and Jane Tugurian.

Dr. Harry Jacobson, Vice Chancellor of Health Affairs of Vanderbilt University, and Dr. John Maupin, President of Meharry Medical College have been constant sources of support.

Many of the patients were seen in the teaching clinic at Saint Thomas Hospital in Nashville. I am indebted to the staff and nurses in the clinic, particularly Joy Smith.

I am indebted to the love and support of my children and their families: Mary Kathleen Meador, Graham K. Meador, Rebecca Meador, Jon and Ann Meador Shayne, Aubrey and Celine Meador, David and Elizabeth Meador Driskill, and Clifton and Mary Neal Meador. My brother Dan has been a steady source of encouragement.

I especially value and appreciate the editing and other assistance from the staff of Vanderbilt University Press: director Michael Ames, Dariel Mayer, Sue Havlish, and Bobbe Needham.

Many physicians have shaped my thinking and have been personal mentors through the years: Robert F. Loeb, Tinsley Harrison, Grant Liddle, David Rogers, Carl Rogers, Joseph Sapira, Stonewall Stickney, Drayton Doherty, H. C. Mullins, and Harry Abram.

Others have shaped my thinking only through their writings. Much of this book comes from their thoughts and ideas. Michael Balint, George Engel, Thomas Kuhn, John Grinder, Richard Bandler, Milton Erickson, Jerome Frank, and Berton Roeuche.

Finally, I want to thank all the patients who taught me so much about people and illness.

# Introduction

The overarching thesis of this book is that the prevailing biomolecular model of disease is too restricted for clinical use.

It took me many years to come to that conclusion. I was pushed to come to that view through my experiences with patients who did not fit the narrow model. Too many exceptions forced me to find an expanded model of disease. These are the stories of those patients and my interaction with them as a physician over a fifty-year period. I have selected patients and their stories that riveted my attention and changed my thinking about the nature of disease, about doctor-patient relationships, and about principles of caring for patients who came to me with symptoms of unknown origin. I have changed the names of the patients and certain other details to preserve their anonymity.

When I graduated from medical school in 1955, I adopted the model of disease then prominent, if not exclusive, in U.S. medicine. It has been called the "biomolecular" model. It is still the dominant model of disease among physicians today. Except for the patient presented in the prologue, the patients' stories in the early chapters of the book illustrate exceptions and aberrations to the narrow biomolecular model. Each case (as I encountered the person and the facts) began to unravel my rigid views about disease and illness. Eventually, I found the biomolecular model of disease applicable only to a narrow segment of patients who seek medical care.

Despite its clinical weaknesses, the restricted biomolecular model remains a powerful biological research tool as we continue to explore the limits of molecular genetics, the genome, and proteomics at the cellular level. We need to draw clear distinctions between the reductionist research model and the need for an expanded clinical model that encompasses the psychological and social aspects of human beings. Human biology and clinical medicine overlap, but they are also quite different and are too often confused.

I did not read Michael Balint until the 1970s. When I did, I was heavily influenced by his writings and began to understand some of the clinical problems I was encountering. Balint studied general practitioners for several years in the United Kingdom as if they were pharmacologic agents. He was examining the correct dosage, underdosage, overdosage, and duration of action of physicians themselves as a drug. Balint developed the term "apostolic function of a physician" to describe the beliefs and teachings of physicians as these affected their relationships with their patients. By "apostolic," he means authoritative teaching.

Of the apostolic function, Balint (1955, 684) writes: "We meant that every doctor has a set of fairly firm beliefs as to which illnesses are acceptable and which are not; how much pain, suffering, fears, and deprivations a patient should tolerate, and when he has the right to ask for help and relief: how much nuisance the patient is allowed to make of himself and to whom, etc., etc. These beliefs are hardly ever stated explicitly but are nevertheless very strong. They compel the doctor to do his best to convert all of his patients to accept his own standards and to be ill or to get well according to them."

Balint goes on to explain the consequences of the doctor's apostolic views.

The effect of the apostolic function on the ways the doctor can administer himself to his patients is fundamental. This effect amounts to always a restriction of the doctor's freedom: certain ways and forms simply do not exist for him, or, if they do exist, somehow they do not come off well and therefore are habitually avoided. This kind of limitation in the way he can use himself is determined chiefly by the doctor's personality, training, ways of thinking, and so on, and consequently has little to do with the actual demands of the case. So it comes about that in certain aspects it is not the patient's actual needs, requirements, and interests that determine the doctor's response to the illnesses proposed to him but the doctor's idiosyncrasies.(Ibid.)

In 1976, Harry S. Abram and I jointly published a chapter in his book *Basic Psychiatry for the Primary Care Physician*. Physicians hardly ever express their beliefs explicitly; nevertheless, Abrams and I modeled our comments along the lines of Balint's thinking and wrote a hypothetical statement in those terms to define and dramatize the narrow biomolecular apostolic function. It is this narrow version under which I had attempted to function during the early years after I graduated from medical school. The hypothetical statement says:

I believe my job as a physician is to find and classify each disease of my patient, prescribe the proper medicine, or recommend the appropriate surgical procedure. The patient's responsibility is to take the medicine I prescribe and follow my recommendations. I believe that man's body and mind are separate and that disease occurs either in the mind or in the body. I see no relationship of the mind to the disease of the body. Medical disease ("real" or "organic" disease) is caused by a single physicochemical defect such as by invasion of the body by a foreign agent (virus, bacterium, or toxin) or from some metabolic derangement arising within the body. I see no patients who fail to have a medical disease. (Abram and Meador 1976, 6)

This is an extreme statement of the biomolecular and single-causation view. I submit that these beliefs are still extant in many medical practices today and that strict application of them is a cause of much of the public's present dissatisfaction with medical care. It was only by an accumulation of confounding clinical experiences, described in the early chapters of this book, that I came to reject the narrow model.

When I was in full-time private practice in Selma, Alabama, in the early 1960s, the senior partner in my practice group got pneumonia. For about three months, I saw all of his patients in addition to my own growing practice. I was surprised to find that many of his patients carried diagnoses of diseases they did not have.

Upon my return to Birmingham and full-time academic life in 1963, I continued to encounter patients who carried diagnoses of nonexistent disease. I wrote a satire called the "Art and Science of Nondisease" and published it in the *New England Journal of Medicine* (Meador 1965). I thought of it as a tongue-in-cheek poke at the foibles of medical practice. The continued responses to that article tell me that I hit on some deep nerve in the way medicine is practiced—that I uncovered some fundamental problem.

I remained puzzled by what to make of this seemingly common error in medical practice until I began to write this book. It is now clear to me that making a false diagnosis of a disease is a consequence of adhering rigidly to the narrow biomolecular model. This view of diseases says, "If a patient has symptoms in the body, then there must be a disease of the body." The physician whose apostolic function demands that he find disease in the body will find disease in the body, whether or not it is real and whether or not it truly explains the patient's symptoms. However, there is not a definable medical disease behind every physical symptom.

In this book, I tell the stories of a series of patients who had symptoms in their bodies but who had no demonstrable medical disease to explain them. Additionally, I raise and explore answers to a set of questions about patients who carry diagnoses of diseases they do not have:

1. How common is the error of assigning a false diagnosis to a patient?
2. If the patient does not have the disease diagnosed, then what does he or she have?
3. What harm can come from having a diagnosis of a disease that is not present?
4. Why has this error been almost completely ignored in the medical literature?

In the later chapters, I present patient stories, findings, and outcomes that came from my adoption of a broader model of disease and illness. Many patients were referred to me by physicians who knew of my interest in problem patients and particularly in patients who carried diagnoses of diseases they did not have.

It is time for a clinical "revolution" or "paradigm shift," to use Thomas Kuhn's terms (Kuhn 1996). In the last chapters of the book, I present applications of a broader paradigm of disease that was proposed by George Engel, which may be a step in this new direction. He suggests the term "biopsychosocial" model (Engel 1977).

By the mid-1970s I had adopted Engel's paradigm. Abram and I formulated the following hypothetical statement to define this broader biopsychosocial model:

I do not believe in a single causation for most diseases. I believe the symptoms of disease arise in a highly complex mix of genetic weakness, psychosocial events and stresses, physicochemical abnormalities, and a host of other factors. I see patients as people with problems who may or may not also have a demonstrable physicochemical defect. If the defect is definable, I prescribe medication aimed at correcting the physio-

logic abnormality or I recommend a surgical procedure. I also
listen to the patient in a manner that will permit him to bring
up whatever is bothering him. I am impressed with the frequency with which my patients can tell me what happened in
their lives just before getting sick. I believe that man's mind
and his body are highly interconnected and related, and that it
is virtually impossible to have disease of one without disease or
some dysfunction of the other. (Abram and Meador 1976, 9)

Balint has said that a physician who wants to delve deeper into
the lives of patients must "undergo a slight but significant change
in personality." Abram and I added that such physicians must also
undergo a considerable "change in [their] belief system."

In the last section of the book, I tell the story of my personal
change, in particular the evolution in how I listened to and observed patients.

I recount my time with Carl Rogers at the Center for the Study
of the Person in La Jolla, California, and with Joseph Sapira, a master clinician at the University of Alabama in Birmingham, and with
Stonewall Stickney, one of my mentors in psychiatry at the University of South Alabama School of Medicine in Mobile. Each taught
me how to listen. I tell the story of watching doctors through one-
way mirrors with H. C. "Moon" Mullins at his family-medicine
teaching clinic in Fairhope, Alabama.

I am suggesting the term "symptoms of unknown origin," or
SUO, for all patients who do not have a ready or immediate medical explanation for their physical symptoms. (I have borrowed from
the well-known term "fever of unknown origin," or FUO.) By using the tentative label SUO, the physician will resist saying the patient is "difficult" or in need of psychiatric treatment. This approach
also avoids the use of more pejorative terms like "crock," "shad," or
"turkey." "Symptoms of unknown origin" is a term that is patently
honest. We really do not know what the origin of any symptom is
when we first meet a patient. All patients initially have symptoms

of unknown origin. My plea is to stay in that mode until the level of certainty of the diagnosis is compelling. This is especially true for patients with chronic or recurring symptoms. Most important, this term enlists the patient in inspecting his or her life to find the variables that may be triggering or even causing the symptoms. In that sense, when appropriately applied, use of the term "SUO" honors the patient's autonomy and frees him or her from unnecessary drugs or procedures and from protracted medical care.

Several colleagues have suggested that the clinical methods described here need a unifying name. They tell me this will help others use, explore, and test the interventions. With that purpose in mind, I suggest the term "physician-directed recollection," or PDR (which also evokes the familiar acronym of the omnipresent *Physicians' Desk Reference*). The mainstay of PDR as a method is enlisting and directing patients to uncover the causes of their symptoms. The physician remains a coach on the sidelines and, through the use of unspecified language and other techniques, calls on the mind of the patient to "re-collect" lost or unknown associations that lie behind the symptoms. The details of the PDR methods are presented in the case reports and in Chapter 20.

# Prologue

The double doors of the amphitheater swung open. A nurse and physician rolled a patient in a wheelchair into the bottom of the amphitheater. A white-haired fiftyish-appearing woman in a bathrobe and nightgown sat slumped to one side of the wheelchair. She was the most pitiful person I had ever seen. Her mouth was half open, with drool dripping from one corner. She struggled to raise her head from its dangling position but could not. Her eyes drooped half closed. It was obvious that the woman was paralyzed.

The rows of seats of the amphitheater slanted upward in an acute angle for nearly two stories. Students sitting in the top rows looked almost directly down into the pit below. Dr. William King, professor of physiology, stood at the bottom of this well with the patient and her physician. Dr. King had just finished his lecture on the biochemistry of the neuromuscular junction. Approaching the end of our physiology course and nearly at the end of our first year of medical school, we were seeing our first patient. We were completing our study of the nervous system. During the first year of medical school, all the focus is on the normal human body—its anatomy, tissues, organs, physiology, and biochemistry. So naturally, as the courses went by, we became more and more interested in seeing live patients—more accurately, we were hungry for clinical contact. The year was 1952.

Dr. King introduced the class to Dr. Sam Riven, the patient's physician and a member of the clinical faculty. Dr. Riven had a busy practice of internal medicine in the community and was widely known as an excellent physician. He looked like a nineteenth-century child's impression of what a doctor should look like. Absent the beard, he reminded me of the physician at the bedside of the sick child in Luke Fildes' classic painting "The Doctor." He wore buttoned suit vest under his long white coat. A Phi Beta Kappa key dangled from a small gold chain that ran from one vest pocket to another. He stood tall and erect and exuded confidence. His hair was graying. There was a trace of a Canadian accent as he spoke in a soft but distinct voice. Dr. Riven introduced Mrs. Gladys Goode to the class and told us this pitiful woman had myasthenia gravis.

Dr. Riven said that Mrs.Goode had agreed to omit one dose of her medicines so we could see how she appeared untreated. The woman made a feeble effort to smile with an ever-so-slight movement of the corners of her mouth; she made a hoarse whispery sound when she tried to speak. He then asked her to perform several tasks. He held up an arm and then let go. The arm flopped back into her lap. She could not move her legs or arms, could not raise her head, could not completely open her eyes. She could barely swallow and could not speak, at least in a voice we could hear. Dr. Riven kept patting her on the head and reassuring her. He repeatedly asked her if she could tolerate a few more minutes. She made a barely noticeable nod of her head. It was more as if she raised her head a fraction of an inch and then let go as her head wobbled a few times on her chest.

Dr. Riven then took a filled syringe from his black bag. He held the syringe high in the air and squirted a small spray from the needle, swabbed the patient's upper arm, and injected the clear liquid into the patient. We sat there in complete silence for several minutes. Slowly the woman began to come alive. There was a science-fiction aura about it—as if Riven was creating life right before our eyes. First she was able to fully open her eyes, then she could close her mouth, then she raised her head to an upright position. The drooling stopped. Slowly she adjusted her position in the wheelchair. And then, like a pure miracle, she sat upright, stood up, spread her arms out to each side, and made a small bow as if to say, "Here I am." We applauded and began talking to each other.

I had sat there amazed. I felt my neck and arms crinkle, as goose bumps rippled across my skin. Awe, in the truest sense of that word, flooded me. For the first time, I had witnessed firsthand the full power of the scientific method. It still amazes me that scientists had identified the details of neuromuscular transmission, isolated and named its chemical compounds, determined the chemical structure of those compounds, identified the biochemical lesion in myasthenia gravis, and then synthesized a drug to counteract the chemical defect that produced the disease. The wonder of the beauty and elegance of that chain of knowledge has never left me.

When the buzz of our talk finally settled down, Mrs. Goode went on to tell us in a clear and strong voice how Dr. Riven had made the diagnosis of myasthenia gravis a year ago and how her life had been brought back nearly to normal by his treating her with physostigmine. Early in the course of her disease, several doctors who had missed the diagnosis had told her she was just neurotic and imagining her weakness. She would be forever grateful to Dr. Riven and was glad to be able to show us medical students what the disease was like. She hoped that she could help to keep us from missing the diagnosis as had happened in her case.

I have practiced and taught medicine for fifty years. I have not made a diagnosis of myasthenia gravis in a single patient, although I have looked for the disease diligently. Even though several people with the disease have been in my practice, I have never made the original diagnosis. It took many years for me to see that myasthenia gravis is a rare disease and that there would be only a few diseases as clearly defined or as dramatically treatable, at least in my lifetime.

The fifty years that have passed since Dr. Riven's demonstration with Mrs. Goode have in no way lessened its impact on me.

The moment Dr. Riven's patient stood up, I knew that I wanted to be able to have that effect on a patient, to be able to find the chemical defect, find the missing hormone, and discover what bacteria or virus had invaded the body. I wanted to make a diagnosis and give the drug or chemical that would precisely correct the biochemical lesion or kill the invading organism. I wanted to do all of that and treat patients and give a normal life back to those who were afflicted.

I thought all diseases would be like myasthenia gravis. I pictured the practice of medicine as finding some missing chemical or element, then supplying the missing substance and curing the patient. I thought all diseases and their remedies would be as straightforward as what I had just witnessed with Dr. Riven. I believed medical science would find similar cures for every single disease and that I would live long enough to make all kinds of diagnoses, give a pill or an injection, and cure people completely. I saw medicine as limitless. What was not curable was only what the sciences had not yet worked out.

During medical school and my postgraduate training, I completely accepted and embraced the biomolecular model of humans and diseases and the virtual separation of mind and body. I thought that the sole job of the physician was to find out what was wrong in the body and fix it. However misguided I might have been, I saw the physician as purely a combination detective and biochemical mechanic of the body. I would live and learn with those narrow notions for several more years to come. I would be a long time in learning that separating the mind from the body imposed clinical restrictions.

The patient stories that follow confronted and forever changed my views about disease and the nature of human beings.

# 1
# An Unlikely Lesson from a Medical Desert

When I drove over the small ridge that had hidden Fort Hood, Texas, from view, my heart sank. As far as I could see, the land stretched into the distance to a faint line of horizon that barely separated sky from ground. I had no idea that such a desolate place would be the setting for one of the most important learning experiences of my medical career.

There were few trees. The entire landscape was pale brown, as though the color green had vanished. Geologically, it was an ancient seabed. Sixty-five million years ago, water had covered the entire area from Fort Hood to the Gulf of Mexico. Giant dinosaur footprints were still visible on the stone riverbeds to the north. I thought at the time that there are some lands too new for human habitation.

The year was 1957. It was the peak of the cold war. The world was poised for a nuclear exchange between the USSR and the United States that thankfully never came. I had just been drafted into the U.S. Army Medical Corps for two years' duty as a general medical officer. The doctor draft had continued after the Korean War, which had ended only a few years before.

The long stretch of bare ground in all directions could not have looked more different from New York City, where I had spent the previous two years in residency training in medicine at Columbia Presbyterian Hospital. The contrast in geography was not the only difference. Instead of treating the sickest patients in New York City, I was to be one of the army physicians who would care for the ten thousand healthy draftees who formed the Fourth Armored Division.

Fort Hood lay about two miles west of Killeen, Texas. The small town's only economic reason for existence was the presence of the army post. Everything about Killeen was tied to the army. There were pawnshops, pool halls, tattoo parlors, hunting and fishing stores, several beer joints, and a few scattered gas stations. Used and repossessed car lots with hundreds of colored triangular flags sat at each end of the town. The highway that ran though the center of Killeen was its business district. It was the highway from Fort Hood to Temple, Texas, twenty-five miles to the east. The treeless residential sections, all new, sprawled across the land in curves of duplexes.

The post hospital sat on the extreme western edge of Fort Hood. Looking out my office window in the dispensary, all I saw was a stretch of land that seemed to reach forever. In the early mornings I often watched the rising columns of dust thrown up by tanks and trucks as they moved slowly out to the impact zone for daily gunnery practice. The armored vehicles eventually disappeared over the horizon, and then all I saw was land and sky. Not only was I geographically isolated, but even worse, I was in medical limbo, banished from medical complexity and challenge.

In my medical training at Columbia Presbyterian Hospital, I saw only the sickest patients or those with complex or rare diseases. The admitting system permitted us to send the less sick patients and those with more common diagnoses to Bellevue or other city hospitals. This process screened out the ordinary illnesses and created a distorted view of medical practice. Medical care is a pyramid with its base in the general population and its tip in referrals and complex diseases. I had been trained to work at the tip of the medical pyramid but had now been assigned to the very bottom. Mostly I would see well soldiers who were suffering from the varied stresses of army duty—too little water (constipation), too much sweating (rashes, jock itch, athlete's feet), too much sun (sunburns), too much marching (blistered and infected feet), and too much weekend liberty (syphilis and gonorrhea).

I was lucky to be assigned to the post hospital. Most of the other drafted doctors were assigned to the various battalions of the Fourth Armored Division spread out across several miles of the post. Each battalion had its own aid station, the site of morning sick call. Whenever the troops were in the field, the battalion doctors had to go with them and live in mock combat conditions. We hospital physicians slept in beds in our own homes and rotated night call at the hospital emergency room. The only thing that determined who was assigned to the hospital and who was assigned to a battalion aid station was length of training before entering the service. Those of us in the hospital had at least one more year of training than the battalion physicians had. That fine difference of one year gave us rank and position at the hospital rather than assignment to the aid stations.

At noon, the battalion surgeons not in the field came to the hospital mess for lunch. These gatherings over lunch became midday rituals. We shared current cases with interesting twists or recalled fascinating patients from our residencies or internships. Often someone described a puzzling finding or a set of symptoms that did not fit into any known diagnosis. Members of the group made suggestions for tests or for specific questions to be asked in the ongoing history. It was a wonderful way to make a dull medical existence more livable—especially for the battalion doctors, who saw only the common results of army duty. They were starved for contact with more serious illnesses, so the informal noon-meal conferences became popular sessions.

Although I worked at the hospital, I also held sick call each morning for the troops assigned to Fourth Armored Division Headquarters. Technically, I was assigned to Headquarters, Headquarters Company, a designation I never understood. There were three doctors and about eight corpsmen at sick call. Each morning a variable number of soldiers would be in line when I arrived. On most days we saw around fifty men, which took about an hour. If there were maneuvers that day, the number could rise to one hundred, making two hours of work. If there was a dress parade on the post, the number could easily exceed two hundred, which took all morning and part of the afternoon. It was our job to see all comers, the sick and the well. It would be my first experience with seeing a patient even close to well since my days in medical school a few years back when we learned to do physicals on our classmates. On sick call, it was our job to separate those who thought they were sick from those who wished they were sick from those who acted sick from those who really were sick.

We had only two placement choices for the soldiers in training—full field duty or admission to the hospital. There was no in-between—no light duty and no way to allow the recruits in training to hang out around the barracks. (The commissioned and noncommissioned officers could go home or lie around the Bachelor Officer's Quarters, the BOQ, until they recovered from minor illnesses or injuries.) The motivation for the recruits to be admitted to the hospital was enormous, however: a soft bed, three hot meals a day, and a nurse or two to look after them. Contrast that with the heat and sweat of long marches, hard bedrolls at night, and cold food. It was no wonder that the number at sick call varied depending on the duties of the day.

We rarely saw anything medically complex among the drafted recruits. Keep in mind that the young men had a physical exam when first drafted that screened out most serious conditions. They had another physical exam on entry into the army before basic training, which screened out what the first process missed or whatever had developed in the meantime. In addition, most of the soldiers were between eighteen and twenty-two years of age, a very healthy period in life. We soon came to realize that we were dealing with an extraordinarily healthy population of young men.

Within a few weeks, I was seriously bored. Other than sick call, I was assigned to the outpatient pediatric department of the hospital. I begged the commanding officer to transfer me to an inpatient unit. I was thankful when he finally assigned me to the female-dependent service. I would be responsible for the care of all hospitalized female dependents on the post. My mornings on sick call were in sharp contrast to my afternoon and evening duty at the hospital, where none of the women had been screened for any disease. There was no prior physical exam to guide me. Any disease was possible and became probable if certain clusters of symptoms were present. My entire thought process had to shift radically from morning sick call, where complex disease was rare, to the afternoon civilian medical care, where anything could appear. Since finding and treating disease was what I had been trained to do, I felt much more at home with the civilians.

It was in the civilian ward that I met the patient who would change forever my views about illness.

At one of our noon gatherings with the battalion physicians, I began to share my problems with this patient. I will call her Amy. She was twelve years old with juvenile-onset diabetes mellitus (now known as type 1 diabetes in contrast to type 2, or adult onset).

Diabetes mellitus was a young internist's dream disease, or so I thought until I met Amy. Diabetes to my mind was the perfect medical disease, somewhat like myasthenia gravis: Some essential chemical (insulin, in this case) is missing from the body; tests (blood glucose levels) can accurately identify the problem; the missing chemical (insulin) can be given; and the patient is cured or at least maintained in a healthy state. Diabetes fit the biomolecular model of disease perfectly. The only job of the physician was to find the offending agent (as in the case of an infection) or the missing chemical (as in the case of a metabolic disorder) and prescribe something to combat the invading organism or replace the missing chemical. The patient, in my limited conception at that time, was only a carrier of the disease.

Amy appeared at one of my afternoon clinics with her mother. She had developed diabetes acutely at age ten, two years before I saw her. At the onset, she abruptly developed diabetic ketoacidosis and had to be rushed to a hospital. Like many juvenile-onset patients, she later went into a partial remission that lasted only a few weeks. During that period she was able to stop all insulin, but the need came back as abruptly as with her onset. She had been taking daily insulin injections for nearly a year when I first saw her.

Her mother also had type 1 diabetes and was quite knowledgeable about management, diet, insulin injections, and the variables that make control of blood sugars possible. In the preceding few months, Amy's control had become extremely unstable. Her mother had already made many adjustments in insulin and diet to no avail.

I relished the challenge of straightening out Amy's clinical state. If there was any disease for which I was fully prepared, it was the treatment and management of diabetes mellitus. Diabetes mellitus had been a special interest of the faculty at Columbia Presbyterian, especially for my chief of medicine, Dr. Robert F. Loeb. Loeb was an authority on the treatment of patients with diabetes, as well as editor of Cecil and Loeb's *Textbook of Medicine,* a leading text of that time. I remember thinking to myself: At last I have a case that I can really get my teeth into. Amy's management would relieve some of the tedium of sick call and the more-or-less routine cases of the other women on my ward.

I spent considerable time reviewing Amy's diet. I moved some food to the afternoon and then a bit to bedtime. I was precise, calculating the grams and calories of carbohydrate, fat, and protein. Dr. Loeb would have been proud of my scientific approach. But none of my changes made any difference. The wild swings in glucose level continued. Amy suffered another episode of ketoacidosis while under what I thought was my most careful observation. I seemed to be having no influence on the disease process.

I changed insulins and altered doses. I tried all the insulin preparations of the day—protamine zinc insulin, Lente, semi Lente, and NPH insulins—adding injections of regular insulin just before meals and at bedtime. All these efforts were to no avail. I tried to get Amy's mother to see a specialist at Scott White Clinic nearby. She refused. I tried to send Amy to Walter Reed Hospital in Washington. She and her mother refused. Her mother kept telling me that they would stick with me, that eventually we would figure out what would work. She was extraordinarily helpful in keeping records and following my advice, but she refused to allow Amy to be referred.

I was spending increasing amounts of time with this patient. I admitted her to the hospital more times than I can recall, at least once every two or three weeks. When she was in ketoacidosis, I felt obligated to stay at her bedside, as I had been trained. The whole affair was becoming a nightmare. My frustration increased week by week. Here was the prototypical medical disease, one for which I had special training. Yet I was failing to make any difference. I had taken every variable into account, but the problem continued, and even got worse.

Our physician lunch group wanted day-by-day reports about Amy. I kept them posted with detailed accounts of her urine and blood tests. I followed several of the group's suggestions for diet or insulin changes. Once we gradually reduced the insulin dose to very low levels and thought we had the problem solved, but the wild fluctuations in her clinical state began again.

The group began to wonder if Amy's mother was up to some bizarre tricks like withholding insulin or upping the dose. I admitted Amy for a prolonged period to test this idea, and the swings in glucose continued even while she was under careful observation in the hospital.

I used everything I had been taught. One member of the group suggested the novel but dangerous idea of putting Amy on small doses of prednisone (a synthetic glucocorticoid compound) so the diabetes would become more severe and therefore somehow more stable and controllable. In my desperation, I actually considered following his advice. It was a dangerous idea, however, and I rejected it.

Then Amy and her mother disappeared. A week went by. Maybe she had switched to one of the other doctors in our group—I asked the group at lunch if anyone had seen her. No one had. I assumed she had finally taken my advice and gone to the Scott White Clinic or to the civilian doctor in town. I felt both relieved and worried. More weeks, then several months, went by, still with no word about Amy. I was puzzled by the lack of a call for her medical records. I wondered if her father had been transferred to another army post. Worst of all, I even began to wonder if she had died.

One day I walked into the waiting room of my afternoon clinic, and there stood Amy and her mother. At first, I held back. But then I saw both were smiling broadly and walking toward me. Both were talking at the same time, excited to tell me where they had been and what had happened. I invited them into my exam area.

The mother quieted Amy with one hand. In a slow and calm voice, she told me what had happened.

Amy had suffered only one hypoglycemic episode in the intervening four months and no episodes of ketoacidosis. Both of them laughed when the mother told me that. I was so puzzled, I said nothing. I was truly dumbfounded. What had I missed? What confounding underlying disease had been discovered? What could possibly produce such a miraculous turnaround?

Amy's mother told me that a new family had moved into the house next door. They had a three-year-old little girl who immediately attracted Amy's attention. From almost the first day, Amy was inseparable from the little girl. To the delight of the young child's mother, Amy did everything for the little girl: changed her clothes, gave her baths, read to her, even fed her. Amy became an adoptive parent. As her mother spoke, Amy smiled and contributed bits of things she liked to do with the girl—riding her on her bike, pulling her in a wagon, and endlessly dressing her in grown-up clothes. It was clear that she was absorbed in the care of the child.

The mother then told me that in addition to the appearance of the little girl, they had given Amy a kitten of her own. Between the little girl and the kitten, Amy's life was filled with joy. Within a week, her diabetes became completely manageable and the wild swings ceased.

The mother said things had been going so well that they had not wanted to bother me anymore. The family was being transferred to another army post, and they wanted to come by and thank me before they left. After a round of questions from me about where they were on insulin dose and diet, I thanked them for coming in and said good-bye.

For some time, I sat at my desk puzzling on the story I had been told. I looked out the window of the dispensary across the vast desert. I could see faintly in the late-afternoon distance a tuft of dust that told me the tanks and trucks were returning. This experience with Amy brought me up short. At first, I assigned the improvement to better adherence to her diet or more careful insulin administration. For a long time, I could not accept the story of the kitten and the young girl and the dramatic turnaround in Amy as anything more than coincidence.

I had been trained to see disease as self-contained, as arising only in the body. Of course patients could be difficult, not take the medicines, participate in activities they should avoid, drink too much, smoke too much, or eat too much. However, all of these were physically describable events related to what patients did or did not do to their bodies. I did not at that time see that the human body could be influenced strongly by the social world around it. In New York, I had seen mostly in-patients with advanced disease, many in the terminal phases. When they left the hospital, I never saw them again. I had no chance to experience the day-by-day influences of living on the disease process. And I certainly did not see that the influences of caring for a little girl and a kitten could affect the action of insulin on glucose metabolism.

It would take many more years for me to accept and begin to use a more systematic and broader view of humans and disease. At the time I was seeing Amy, I still saw the mind and body as two separate systems. Disease was either medical-physical and therefore "real," or it was mental-emotional and therefore "not real." Amy was the first patient to show me vividly that the human mind and body are not separable. Further, the internal physiological world and the external social world for each of us are quite connected. More important, the social connections and their power can be unique for each patient.

I also had to accept the idea that I had become part of Amy's external world—that I probably had contributed my own anxieties to Amy's problems. She most certainly had done better without me than she had when I was seeing her regularly. I would learn years later that doctors can unwittingly assist in making or keeping people sick, just as they can assist them to improve. The placebo effect works in both directions. None of these broader thoughts occurred to me while I was at Fort Hood.

# 2
# Texas Heat

During the winter after I arrived at the hospital at Fort Hood, I kept seeing a young soldier ambling down one of the long corridors. He slid his hand along the wall as he shuffled along aimlessly, pausing from time to time to stare out a window. He had the look of one of those zombies from a 1930s black-and-white horror movie. He never acknowledged me or spoke or even looked like he knew where he was going.

I asked Red McGregor, my ward sergeant (who knew everything about the hospital—and the U.S. Army, for that matter) what he knew about this soldier I kept seeing in the hallways. Red had been a combat medic in Korea and stayed in the army after the war. The summer before, Red told me, they had brought the soldier in from the field unconscious and with a temperature of 106 degrees. Summers in West Texas begin early and run late; the heat is merciless. The soldier clearly had a heat stroke but unfortunately there was a delay in treating him in the field and even after he got to the hospital. The usual treatment in the field was to strip off all the clothing of anyone even suspected of having a heat problem and then to douse them with water and ice if available. When they got to the hospital, the ice was continued and every effort was made to reduce the body's temperature as quickly as possible. Heat stroke is a true medical emergency. Minutes count if brain damage is to be avoided.

Red said they were too late on both ends of the treatment with this young soldier. He suffered severe brain damage. The behavior I had noticed was its outward expression. Apparently he was showing some improvement, but the residual damage was severe. He had little memory and could not do simple arithmetic or even follow a series of simple commands. From time to time, he would get loose from his ward and wander around the halls until someone brought him back. He was finally discharged severely impaired with full medical disability.

The tragic case rightfully set the commanding general's teeth on edge: In the future, any field commander who had even one case of heat injury would be brought before general courts martial and punished if found guilty of neglect of his troops. The definition of neglect was merely the occurrence of a single case of heat injury. The reason for this severe injunction was that heat injury of any sort was 100 percent preventable. If a commander looked after his troops, heat injury should not occur.

There are two forms of heat injury: heat exhaustion and heat stroke. Heat exhaustion is caused from loss of salt (sodium chloride) from excessive sweating and too little replacement of the salt combined with drinking too much water. The body becomes dilute with reference to salt; if this state continues, convulsions can occur. Usually the victim develops extreme fatigue and muscle cramps as the first symptoms. The state is easily prevented by taking salt tablets and being careful not to drink too much water without some salt intake. (Since then, salt tablets have been eliminated and replaced with dilute salt-containing liquids such as Gatorade.) The treatment is replacement of the salt either orally if there is no emergency or intravenously if the situation is severe.

Heat stroke is quite a different syndrome. For reasons not known in 1957, a person after prolonged exposure to high temperature in the environment would suddenly stop sweating. With this major route for losing heat from the body through evaporation cut off, the body temperature can and often does rise to extraordinarily high levels, even as high as 106 to 108 degrees. These high temperatures cause brain injury and death if not rapidly corrected. Prevention is essential. Prevention requires a person to move from the sun to the shade for at least ten minutes out of every hour and to completely cease all physical activity for the full ten-minute period.

The tragic single case from the year before had the entire post on constant alert. Each field unit carried water, salt tablets (now no longer recommended), and ice in trucks, ready in case anyone complained of any symptom related to heat. At the hospital dispensary where we worked and saw sick call in the mornings, there were three large bathtubs and a huge ice machine capable of producing several large bags of crushed ice in a few minutes. As soon as any field unit called in announcing the transport of someone suspected of heat injury, the entire staff of the dispensary and all medical officers went into high gear. I knew this because we repeatedly ran heat-stroke drills. The drills involved every unit on the base at one time or another, so I saw the ice machines in action on several occasions as corpsmen hauled mock heat injuries to the dispensary. As soon as the tubs were filled with ice cubes, the corpsmen dumped in several gallons of brine. It was cold enough to make ice cream, as one of the men put it.

Not too long after the fort was in full alert for the upcoming heat season, the first case occurred. Red grabbed me as we headed down the long corridor to the dispensary. He mumbled as we ran toward the emergency room, "There won't be just one. Never are." The remark struck me as unusual.

Red and the rest of the group and I stood on the loading dock out in back of the dispensary. We saw three large trucks coming in a cloud of dust in the distance. "Radio just said there was ten of 'em," Red said to the group. "I knew it'd be more than one. Always is."

The trucks all backed up to the loading dock and we began unloading limp soldiers. When they arrived, all ten were unconscious, limp, and naked, having been stripped in the field. Red, as senior medic, took charge. Rather than sort them out and take temperatures, the corpsmen and the rest of us started dumping the men into the ice-and-brine tubs we had prepared before the trucks arrived at the dispensary. We had to put two and three to a tub. Two of the men became conscious before we could put them into the ice bath. Within a few seconds after we put the other men into the brine, they started yelling and trying to get out. In a few minutes, we sorted out the one man who truly had some degree of heat injury. He lay limp for several more minutes before moving at all. The other nine were sitting around the dispensary tub room shivering from the ice bath. Fortunately, the one injured man had only a mild elevation of temperature and suffered no detectable brain injury.

Red said that was nearly always the way it went. The brine test never failed to make the diagnosis.

The master sergeant who brought the men in described what appeared to be a mass occurrence of fainting. First one man slumped to the ground, followed in quick succession by the other nine. In the opinion of the sergeant, some of the men were genuinely unconscious. He suspected two were faking it. He had tested them in the field by pinching them and trying to get a response to pain. Eight had showed no response to pain until we put them into the brine. The response even then was a bit sluggish, taking a few moments for all the men to rouse. When they did, they became insistent about getting out of the tubs. Most of them just jumped out—blue lipped and shivering from the extreme cold of the mixture.

I was puzzled by this sympathetic reaction. As best I could put the story together, one man went down with heat injury. The other men, seeing him go down, believed the conditions were severe enough to cause heat injury. Already feeling the effects of heat, as everyone in the field (especially the young recruits) did when the temperature got high enough, they somehow reacted by losing consciousness, apparently believing that they too were suffering from heat injury. Of course, a few probably faked it.

When we finished icing the men, an old corpsman from the field confirmed Red's observation. He told me he had seen this kind of multiple occurrence of sympathetic fainting before. He also pointed to the multiple episodes of fainting that frequently occur when soldiers stand at parade rest too long. He believed that one faint would trigger a sequence of fainting. "Either you have no faintings or you will have a lot of faintings. There's no in-between," is the way he put it.

"Just like with heat cases," Red echoed. "Some of 'em aren't faking either. I don't know what to call it. Maybe it's like hypnosis or something. The mind's a powerful thing."

I wondered about those soldiers and their sympathetic loss of consciousness from time to time over the years. This was one more small but unexplained crack in the strict biomolecular model of man. I filed the episode somewhere in my subconscious mind along with other accumulating bits of unexplained phenomena. "Cognitive dissonance," a phrase tossed around then, is what I learned to call these unresolved bits. I was becoming aware of my propensity for keeping cognitive dissonance alive and unreconciled in my mind.

There is a phenomenon beyond the biomolecular model that I will call "sympathetic illness." I saw it firsthand with the heat cases. The phenomenon of sympathetic illness occurs from time to time in civilian medicine, sometimes in epidemic proportions. The heat cases fascinated me—not because I understood their meaning, but because I did not.

# 3
# Dr. Drayton Doherty and Miss Cootsie

In 1961, I joined a multispecialty-practice group in Selma, Alabama, a town of about thirty thousand people. I would be the junior member of the group and the only internist and endocrinologist— the others were surgeons, general practitioners, and one obstetrician/gynecologist. The senior partner was Dr. Drayton Doherty, the surgeon who had delivered me into the world by cesarean section in 1931. I was the second new doctor to come to town since World War II. The medical scientific gulf between doctors trained before and those trained after World War II was wide and nearly unbridgeable.

Although my dream was academic medicine, I had run out of money. At that time, academic medicine paid salaries of around three thousand dollars a year. With a wife and two young sons, I needed income. I accepted an offer to join Dr. Doherty and his group. My contracted salary in practice offered nine thousand dollars a year, the going rate for internists in 1961. I would practice medicine and see where life led me.

For getting a jump-start in my practice, I could not have been luckier. In the first week, I was asked to see and treat the wife of the probate judge. Irene Johnson, I will call her, had been one of the social leaders of the county, full of life and wit and loved by nearly everyone. She had been an avid bridge player. Over the preceding few years, she had slipped into a reclusive life. She had stopped driving her car and rarely left her home. According to the rumors around town, she had become mentally retarded. As the new young doctor who had trained Up East, I was asked to see her in consultation.

When I first laid eyes on Irene Johnson, I knew immediately what the problem was. She had lost most of her hair, and what was left was sparse and brittle. Her lips were thick and protuberant. She looked pale and waxen. Her skin was coarse and thick and felt like fine sandpaper. Her lids drooped halfway over her eyes. She spoke very slowly and with a husky deep voice. Her deep tendon–reflex relaxation time was long and slow. I had never seen a more severe case of untreated hypothyroidism, which I confirmed with a protein-bound iodine level and a radioiodine uptake. I had just set up the first nuclear medicine laboratory in Selma. I did the first radioiodine study in the region on Irene Johnson.

I don't know who was luckier, the patient or I. To have a curable disease like hypothyroidism in one of your first patients is like a dream come true. To have a hypothyroid patient who is famous locally and well known to have "lost her mind and will" is nearly unbelievably lucky. I cannot imagine a quicker way to build a practice. How the diagnosis had been missed for so long is still a puzzle to me. I suppose the development of the clinical state was so slow and insidious that it was just not seen as a change. I also discovered there was a widespread misconception about what hypothyroid patients looked like. Whatever the reasons for missing the diagnosis, everyone thought Irene Johnson was senile and demented and "just rapidly aging."

With the administration of thyroid extract, the transformation in Irene Johnson was dramatic and miraculous. She regrew a full head of hair. Her skin returned to a silky texture and all the puffiness of her eyes and face went away. She emerged—a metamorphosis from another life form. Within a few months, she returned to a fully active social life, was able to drive her car, and soon was again beating everyone at bridge. She had not been actually demented but was mentally very slow from her hypothyroid state. Even when she was hypothyroid, she was mentally accurate but just slow in responding. Few people waited for her slow responses. Once back to normal and out on the town, she could not tell enough people in a day what a terrific doctor I was. She was a walking, talking, visible advertisement for my practice, which grew rapidly. I was soon engulfed, the target of every patient who had been misdiagnosed or mistreated or misunderstood or who had done poorly, although I never had another medical home run quite like Irene Johnson.

No disease on earth is more treatable than hypothyroidism. It is the king of biomolecular diseases and one of science's crowning achievements. Early scientists discovered the thyroid gland by anatomic dissections of cadavers. They much later discovered that removal of the thyroid gland in animals led to identifiable metabolic changes: Metabolism slowed. Then in the 1800s, the clinical state of hypothyroidism was described in humans when autopsies of patients showing an absence of the thyroid gland. Eventually, reversal of the hypothyroid state was achieved by ingestion of the ground-up thyroid glands of pigs and cows. Many years later, the active agent was chemically determined to be thyroxine, later to be tri-iodothyronine. Before the chemical formula of the thyroxine molecule could be discovered, the entire atomic theory of matter and the complete periodic table of mineral elements had to be discovered and described, with the atomic weights of each identified and defined. The empirical formula of the thyroxine molecule was found to be $C_{15} H_{10} I_4 N NaO_4x H_20$, with a molecular weight of 798.86.

When I wrote that prescription for thyroid extract for Irene Johnson, I was standing on the shoulders of thousands of scientists who came before me. Each scientist drilled a bit deeper into the puzzle of the thyroid gland until finally we could make a synthetic molecule of thyroxine, give that tiny molecule to patients, and bring them back to physical normalcy. I remain in awe of the scientific method and the reductionistic method of inquiry that has led us to understand smaller and smaller components of nature.

I want to make it as clear as I possibly can that this book is not a criticism of scientific reductionism. I am in awe of the method and its effectiveness. My point here is that scientific reduction is not the same process as clinical medicine.

It is the sheer scientific power of the biomolecular model that has blinded so many as to its clinical limitations and restrictions. Irene Johnson's hypothyroidism was pure biochemistry out of control, and her cure was purely biochemical.

♦ ♦ ♦

Over the years in private practice, Dr. Doherty and I got to be close and good friends, and he was delighted to see my practice take off so rapidly. Like other doctors trained before World War II, he was weak in the advances that science had brought into clinical medicine. He called on me often with troublesome patients. Although he was an excellent technical surgeon, Dr. Doherty's clinical notions were mostly out of date. He continued to use unnecessary flax poultices on his post-op patients. He often prescribed toxic strychnine and used inert tonics and gave a lot of unneeded vitamins. He spoke of ill-defined stimulants and stomatics and often still used calomel to purge the bowels of his patients. His practice was from another time and place and it bothered me intellectually, although I never told him directly. He was just not scientific enough for my taste at that time, even though I respected him as a friend and father figure. But he had two skills that I have seen no physician match. He was completely accurate on assessing acute surgical abdomens, and he could listen to and understand people.

♦ ♦ ♦

One day Dr. Doherty asked me to see a longtime patient of his. Looking back, I would wonder if he had some object lesson in mind when he asked me to see her. Maybe this was his way of putting me in my place. Her name was Frances Conrad, but she was known affectionately to everyone for miles around as Miss Cootsie.

Dr. Doherty could barely suppress a grin when he asked me to take over her care. If I was riding high on the results of curing Irene Johnson's hypothyroidism, I would plummet to a new low from what was about to happen with Miss Cootsie.

Miss Cootsie was eighty-five years old and a legend in the medical community. Her son was a prominent businessman in town and he had asked Dr. Doherty if the "young doctor who had cured Mrs. Johnson" could see his mother. Dr. Doherty had jumped at the opportunity and volunteered me immediately. He told me he could not wait for me to see Miss Cootsie.

Miss Cootsie was a well-known invalid and, like so many invalids, was seen as very weak and lacking the stamina required for the rigors of an office visit. She required a house call, no matter what the problem. About the only time invalids left their homes was for occasional Sunday afternoon automobile rides around town. Even then, they wore their bathrobes and gowns.

Miss Cootsie lived upstairs in a large antebellum house in town with Little Cootsie, her spinster daughter, who was in her sixties. The first floor of the house had been shut down for use, for reasons I never discovered. All the furniture downstairs was covered in white cloths. As I had been instructed by Dr. Doherty, I wound my way up the stairs to Miss Cootsie's bedroom at the front of the house and called out her name. Little Cootsie had an adjoining bedroom. A bath, added years before, now served as a combination kitchen and bath. Miss Cootsie was sitting in a rocking chair looking out the front window onto the lawn and street below. She had a commanding view of nearly two blocks in both directions.

When I walked into the room, it was immediately apparent that Miss Cootsie had the largest goiter I have ever seen. It hung down like a strange bib over her upper chest. It was the size of a grapefruit and it bobbed slightly with each heartbeat. There was no subject in endocrinology for which I was better prepared than the understanding and treatment of goiters. Here I was standing in front of the most magnificent goiter I had ever seen. I was really going to be famous when I shrank that goiter with medicine. If Irene Johnson's recovery from hypothyroidism had built my practice, the shrinkage of Miss Cootsie's famous goiter without surgery would just explode it. I would be famous for miles around. I have to admit that I had oceanic visions of grandeur.

Miss Cootsie quickly told me she had outlived three previous doctors before she took on Dr. Doherty. She told me she had refused repeated offers of surgery for her goiter and that she would refuse surgery from me. She had an air of pure defiance about her and reminded me of Lionel Barrymore in one of his sterner roles. The workup in those days for thyroid disease was meager, but by those measures her overall thyroid hormonal function was normal. Her physical examination was also normal, as were her routine blood tests, which I drew and took back to the clinic lab.

There were many series of articles in the literature of the 1960s about patients with goiters that had been shrunk with the administration of thyroid extract (thyroxin was not yet available). The theory was that the added thyroid hormone suppressed the pituitary secretion of thyroid-stimulating hormone, and without this stimulus for growth, the goiter would go away. I began Miss Cootsie on a small dose of thyroid extract, planning to increase the dose gradually. I would come by to see her again in two weeks, I told her.

Late one night, just before the two weeks were up, I got a call from the sheriff. Miss Cootsie was outside her house in her underwear running up and down the street. Apparently she had gone stark, raving insane. The sheriff was there to help Little Cootsie find her mother. I got over to the house, helped the sheriff and Little Cootsie catch Miss Cootsie, got her into the car, and drove her out to the hospital. Miss Cootsie was clearly hyperthyroid and wild, talking as fast as her mouth and lips would move. Little Cootsie said her mother tripled the dose of thyroid I ordered and may have taken the whole bottle. As soon as I got her into the hospital, she went into acute heart failure with pulmonary edema. Within a day of clearing the pulmonary edema, while she was still psychotic she developed pneumonia. A few days later, as she was beginning to clear mentally, she developed a penicillin reaction with a violent rash that covered her entire body. Three long months later, I finally got her back home and off all drugs and back to her baseline with a huge goiter.

I learned my lesson: Invalids should be accepted and tolerated, even if they have a large goiter. Whatever reasons drove them to become invalids in the first place are best left alone. Some people have a deep need to play the sick role. On all my subsequent house calls, I just sat and listened to Miss Cootsie tell me about everybody who had passed on the street below. In addition, she described in great detail her constant and continuing problems with her irregular bowel habits. I listened, but I still could not take my eyes off her huge goiter.

I had learned the hard way that what goes up must come down. The heights of success with Irene Johnson were balanced by the low of the clinical defeat with Miss Cootsie. To this day, I would swear Dr. Doherty somehow knew I would learn my lesson from Miss Cootsie. He had me tell him the story over and over in the lounge, as he doubled over with laughter.

# 4
# All Some Patients Need Is Listening and Talking

One day Dr. Doherty said, "You know, medicine is very different now from when I came along. I see you do things that I barely understand. In my early days, we really didn't have a whole lot to offer medically. Let me tell you a story that might help you understand what I mean."

In the spring of 1938, Dr. Doherty admitted a sixty-year-old black man to the black hospital. The small, completely segregated hospital was located at the edge of town in an old house that had been converted into a fifteen-bed hospital. Six of the beds were located upstairs at the rear of the house in what had previously served as a sleeping porch. The patient was admitted to that porch.

Dr. Doherty went on to tell me that the patient (I will call him Vance Vanders) had been ill for many weeks and had lost a large amount of weight, estimated to be fifty or more pounds. He looked extremely wasted and near death. His eyes were sunken and resigned. The clinical suspicions in those days for anyone with a wasting disease were either tuberculosis or widespread cancer. Repeated tests and chest x-rays for both these diseases were negative, as was the physical examination. Despite a nasogastric feeding tube, Vance Vanders continued on a downhill course, refusing to eat and vomiting whatever was put down the tube. He said repeatedly he was going to die, and he soon reached a stage of near stupor. Drifting in and out of consciousness, he was barely strong enough to talk. Only then did his wife, who had stayed by his bedside, ask to talk to Dr. Doherty privately. Dr. Doherty knew both Vanders and his wife personally. Both worked on the farm of an acquaintance of Dr. Doherty.

The sick man's wife appeared extremely nervous and anxious. She made Dr. Doherty swear never to tell anyone the story she was about to tell.

Here was what Vance Vanders's wife told Dr. Doherty: About four months before Vanders was admitted to the hospital, he had a run-in with the local witch doctor or "priest," as he was called. It was well known that many blacks of the area practiced voodoo and that there were several priests in the region. Late one night, a priest had summoned Vanders to the cemetery. The wife had not been able to uncover why he called Vanders, only that an argument occurred. While they were arguing, the priest waved a bottle of some foul-smelling liquid about Vanders's face. The priest told Vanders that he had "voodooed" him and that Vanders would die in the very near future, that there was no way out, and that even the medical doctors could not save him. Vanders was doomed to die. He staggered home that evening and did not eat again. Several weeks later, he was admitted to the small hospital in a moribund state.

Neither the wife nor Vanders had come forward to tell the story because the voodoo priest had told them he would voodoo all their children and as many other people as it took to keep them silent. Terrified, especially since they had seen Vanders's illness unfold as predicted, the couple kept the story to themselves. Now that Vanders was near death, his wife came forward to tell Dr. Doherty in hopes that he could somehow miraculously save her husband.

Dr. Doherty said he was puzzled but fascinated by the story. Knowing that Vanders was very near death, he spent a lot of time that night thinking about what approach he should take. Whatever he did, he knew it had to be done right away or Vanders would certainly die.

The next morning, with his plan in mind, Dr. Doherty came to

Vanders's bedside. He had asked that all the kin be present. Ten or more of them gathered in the six-bed ward. They were trembling and frightened to be associated with this doomed man. They pulled away from the bed as Dr. Doherty approached.

Dr. Doherty announced in his most authoritative voice that he now knew exactly what was wrong with Vanders. He told them of a harrowing encounter at midnight the night before in the local cemetery, where he had lured the voodoo priest on some false pretense. Dr. Doherty said he told the priest that he had uncovered his secret voodoo and found out precisely how he had voodooed Vanders. At first, the priest had laughed at him. Dr. Doherty said he choked the priest against a tree nearly to death until the priest described exactly what he had done to Vanders.

Here is what Dr. Doherty told Vanders and the small crowd of kin who had gathered around the bed. (He told me they hung on every word he uttered.) "That voodoo priest rubbed some lizard eggs into your stomach and they climbed down into your real stomach and hatched out some small lizards. All but one of them died, leaving one large one which is eating up all your food and the lining of your body. I will now get that lizard out of your system and cure you of this horrible curse."

With that, he summoned the nurse. She had, by prearrangement, filled a large syringe with apomorphine (a powerful injectable emetic). With great ceremony, Dr. Doherty pointed the syringe to the ceiling and inspected it most carefully for several moments. He squirted the smallest amount of clear liquid into the air and lunged toward Vanders. The patient by now had gathered enough strength to be sitting up wide-eyed in the bed. He pressed himself against the headboard, trying to escape the injection. Dr. Doherty with dramatic motions pushed the needle into Vanders's arm and delivered the full dose of apomorphine. With that he wheeled about, said nothing, and dramatically left the ward.

In a few minutes, the nurse reported that Vanders was beginning to vomit. When Dr. Doherty arrived at the bedside, Vanders was retching, one wave of spasms after another. His head was buried in a metal basin that sat on the bed. After several minutes of continued vomiting and at a point judged to be near its end, Dr. Doherty pulled from his black bag, artfully and secretly, a green lizard. At the height of the next wave of retching, he slid the lizard into the basin. He called out in a loud voice, "Look, Vance, look what has come out of you! You are now cured. The voodoo curse is lifted!"

There was mumbling across the room. Several relatives fell on the floor and began to moan. According to Dr. Doherty and the nurse who witnessed the event, Vanders saw the lizard through his squinted eyes, did a double take, and then jumped back to the head of the bed, his eyes wide and his jaw hanging open. He looked dazed. He did not vomit again but drifted into a deep sleep within a minute or two, saying nothing. His pulse rate was very slow (the exact count was not recalled), and his breathing became slow and extremely deep. This sleep/coma lasted more than twelve hours, into the next morning. When he woke, Vanders was ravenous. He gulped down large quantities of milk, bread, some meat, and eggs before he was made to stop for fear he would rupture his stomach.

Within a week, Vanders was discharged. Within a few weeks, he had regained his weight and strength. He lived another ten or more years, dying of what sounded like a heart attack, having no further encounter with the voodoo priest. No one else in the family was affected.

I knew the nurse who had witnessed the events. She confirmed Dr. Doherty's story. My uncle, Dr. Sam Kirkpatrick Sr., a local physician, also confirmed it, as did the farmer on whose land Vanders worked.

I did not know what to make of this strange and fascinating story. It was my first encounter with hexing and voodoo. Initially, I dismissed the tale as a superstitious display of primitive ignorance. But it was evident that Vanders believed at the deepest level that he was cursed and doomed to die. I wondered how words could be so powerful that they can induce death. Can just words, mere words, have that power? It was a completely new concept to me—almost beyond belief. That was why I kept asking others to verify the story, and they did. Eventually I had to accept the story as true. I could not find a hole or crack in it.

In some equally inexplicable way, Dr. Doherty had been able to reverse what was almost certain to be a fatal outcome. He had done it with actions and words. He had made up a story that was both plausible and believable in the extraordinarily strange voodoo world of Vanders. Dr. Doherty was able to enter this world completely. His words and actions convinced Vanders that he was healed. Once convinced, Vanders became well.

Dr. Doherty wanted me to know that there was a lot more to being a physician than measuring chemicals in blood and urine and prescribing drugs. He said, "Clifton, all some people need is some listening and talking."

• • •

Thirty years later, I finally published the story of Vanders in "Hex Death: Voodoo Magic or Persuasion" (Meador 1992a), in which I drew a parallel between voodoo/hex death and the diagnosis of cancer in some people and in a patient of mine. This man died not from cancer but from *believing* he was dying of cancer. I also participated in the report of this case by the BBC in a program called "Placebo" on the Discovery Health TV Channel in January 2003.

I included in my report Walter Cannon's observations on the phenomenon of hex death in primitive cultures. Cannon, a renowned physiologist at Harvard, reported several hex deaths observed by Westerners in primitive cultures around the globe. Poisoning was ruled out as carefully as possible.

Cannon reported that there are three essential elements in a successful hex death:

1. The victim, all acquaintances, and family members must accept the ability and power of the witch doctor to induce death by hexing.
2. With no exceptions, all known previous victims of hexing must have died.
3. Everyone known to the victim, including parents and friends, must begin to act as though the victim were already dead.

Cannon (1957) accepted hex death as a documented phenomenon worthy of further scientific inquiry.

The biomolecular model is so pervasive that unless one can posit a possible molecular explanation for a phenomenon, the subject is excluded from research. In other words, until the molecular basis is known, no phenomenon exists. Examples of "nonphenomena" excluded from research are death by hexing, religious conversion, persuasion, hypnotism, trance induction, the placebo effect and its opposite, the nocebo effect, much of human behavior, and most psychosocial influences on disease (Frank and Frank 1991).

The biomolecular model for biological research is still far from exhausted as we move into the details of the genome, proteomics, and genetic transmission. The exceptions I have listed here exist at the individual or social level and are outside the molecular sphere. All are phenomena that bear on clinical medicine and the care of sick people. All deserve scientific exploration by nonmolecular techniques.

# 5
# Diagnoses
# Without Diseases

In 1962, Dr. Doherty developed pneumonia and had to be away from his practice for several months. He asked me to take over the medical patients he had been following. The experience was an eye-opener.

Many of his patients did not have the diseases that Dr. Doherty had diagnosed. In fact, many did not have any medically defined disease I could document. They had lots of symptoms but no medical disease.

Some carried diagnoses of pernicious anemia and were receiving injections of vitamin $B_{12}$ every month. It was the correct treatment for pernicious anemia but for the wrong patients and the wrong reason. The Schilling test had just come out, and it could measure the ability of the gut to absorb radioactive $B_{12}$. I set up the test in our clinic's new Nuclear Medicine Laboratory and soon we were making measurements. None of Dr. Doherty's patients with a diagnosis of pernicious anemia had any problem absorbing vitamin $B_{12}$. In fact, less than a handful of patients from all the practices we tested with the Schilling test had abnormal results. A lot of patients were being treated with $B_{12}$ injections for pernicious anemia, but only a few had the disease.

What was even more remarkable to me was that none of Dr. Doherty's patients seemed at all delighted when I told them the test was normal and they could stop taking the $B_{12}$ injections. The most common response was something like this: "Well, let's just wait until Dr. Doherty gets well and let's see what he says about all this. Now just go ahead and give me that vitamin shot. It makes me feel so good."

Naively, I had thought some would say, "Oh, Doctor, thank you so much for telling me I don't have that disease. Now I can stop taking those vitamin shots every month." Not a single patient told me that. I was waking up to the real world.

Dr. Doherty had a number of patients with "emphysema" who had normal timed vital capacities when I tested them in our new pulmonary function laboratory that I had set up. Others had diagnoses of rheumatoid arthritis with negative tests and findings for the disease. "Low blood sugar" was one of Dr. Doherty's favorite diagnoses. Many of the diagnoses had no counterpart in contemporary medical terminology. Examples of these were "weak kidneys," "spastic colon," "dropped kidneys," "retroverted or tilted uterus," "hiatus hernia," and just "stomach trouble." "Sinus trouble" covered nearly any complaint above the neck.

Not only did many of the patients fail to have the diagnosis given them by Dr. Doherty, they did not have any diagnosable medical disease that I could find. They were, nearly to a person, medically healthy. Yet they had myriad physical symptoms and complaints. Only a few seemed pleased to be told they did not have their diseases. Dr. Doherty's power to convey diagnoses of diseases the patients did not have was greater than my ability to persuade them they did not have any diseases.

I was puzzled by the meaning of all of this. I was also conflicted about how to handle these diagnoses of nonexistent diseases. On one hand, I felt a strong obligation to be honest with the patients, but on the other hand, I felt uncomfortable counteracting much of Dr. Doherty's practice. He had found a system that worked for him—giving a diagnosis, no matter how far-fetched, was for him the best way to handle these patients with multiple symptoms. At some fundamental level, I recoiled from this approach.

Fortunately, I could avoid the conflict with Dr. Doherty. He soon returned to his practice, and I had accepted an appointment on the faculty at the University of Alabama at the School of Medicine in Birmingham. I could leave the problem behind me. I am not sure how I would have handled it if I had stayed.

• • •

If there is a clinical heaven, in Birmingham I was finally back in it. Returning to academic medicine for me was like oxygen to a winded runner or water to a man lost in a desert. Teaching and seeing complex clinical problems was what I wanted to do.

My official job at the School of Medicine at the University of Alabama was to run the N.I.H. Clinical Research Center, set up a system to review research applications, and provide clinical care and oversight to the patients in the research center. I spent most of my time teaching medical students, residents, and fellows in endocrinology and seeing patients referred to the medical center with possible endocrine problems.

There were only four trained endocrinologists in the entire state of Alabama, and we were all at the medical center in Birmingham. Together we saw examples of every conceivable endocrine disease known at that time. There was no such specialty then as pediatric endocrinology, so we saw the full spectrum of life—babies, children, and adults. Within a few years, I had seen examples of not only every recognized endocrine disorder but also nearly every known variation. There will never be such a concentration of endocrine diseases again. This was the era when subspecialists existed only in large academic medical centers. In the years to follow, other endocrinologists moved into clinical practice and built their own private practices, eventually diluting the population that was referred to the medical center. This was the golden era, and we saw it all.

Endocrinology was one of the first specialties in medicine to become truly scientific. We could measure what we talked about.

That had great appeal to me. We lived during the transition from urine measurements using animal/mice assays, or analyses, to very precise direct measurements of hormones in blood. The advent of highly sensitive radioimmunoassays and paper chromatography expanded our ability to measure very small quantities of nearly every hormone. These new tools allowed us to measure at the nanogram level, an astounding nine decimal places out from one gram— 0.000000001—a great achievement in method. In a short time, the exact definitions for diagnosing low and high levels of hormones were rewritten.

Making a diagnosis of an endocrine disorder became extraordinarily precise. We could measure not only the level of hormones but also the pituitary-stimulating hormones that regulated many of the hormone levels and secretions. The negative feedback system then permitted extremely refined definitions of excesses or deficiencies of the major hormones. Excesses shut off, and deficiencies produced, high levels of the pituitary-stimulating hormones. Medicine could not get too scientific for me, and I was living and practicing on the cutting edge of clinical science.

As we took these new ideas and tools out into our talks to the county medical societies, our referral practice at the medical center mushroomed. As soon as we described and taught the doctors across the state what to look for, we began to see referred examples in Birmingham. We began to publish reports of individual cases, collections of patients, and unusual examples of the various endocrine disorders.

Along with all the endocrine and metabolic disorders we saw in the referred patients, there was a steady stream of patients who had no endocrine or metabolic disorder. Many of these patients already carried a diagnosis of one or more medical diseases that they often did not have. It soon became apparent to me that Dr. Doherty had not been alone in his free use of medical diagnoses when no diseases were present. I found this a widespread pattern.

The patients I saw had been referred because their doctors

could not make a diagnosis to explain the entire clinical picture. Often there were diagnoses of nonexistent diseases, but even those failed to explain the picture. I also found it a common pattern with complex patients for doctors to be saying to themselves, "Well, maybe it's metabolic," or "Well, maybe it's endocrine." Metabolic and endocrine diseases were both at that time a bit beyond the edge of common practice. Both fields were very new, being defined and described almost month by month. Even the defined metabolic or endocrine disorders sounded a bit obscure and even mystical. Whatever the reasons, we saw many patients with the referring note, "Could this be a metabolic or endocrine problem?"

I could not bring myself to do what other specialists tended to do. I often saw notes that said, "No Gyn problem in this patient"; or, "I can find no evidence for cardiac disease"; or, "There is no solid evidence for GI disease." In other words, the specialist would focus on the specialty area only and clear the patient of any problem in that area. This was an honest and direct approach. I intend no criticism of that method. I just could not bring myself to use it. Beyond all my attraction to the biochemical sciences of medicine, a patient was sitting there with symptoms I could not explain with my measurements or observations.

It was relatively easy, given our increasingly accurate measurements, to say, "No metabolic or endocrine problem found." That still left me with patients loaded with symptoms, complaining, and in real distress, describing lives of misery and pain and discomfort. They called up the general doctor in me.

I was not aware of it at the time, but I was about to become engaged in the mind-body dichotomy. This false dichotomy is still very much alive and functioning today, but at that time it was deeply entrenched in medical practice. The unwritten but nearly absolute rule, if written, would have gone something like this: "There are diseases of the body and there are diseases of the mind. If no disease is found in the body, then there must be a disease of the mind. The mind and the body are completely separate and there is no connection. Patients either have a disease of the mind or they have a disease of the body."

The unwritten rule of this false dichotomy went a bit further: "Given a patient with physical symptoms and no findings of disease in the body, the patient has a disease of the mind." There was (and still is in some circles today) the heavy implication that the patient was making up the symptoms—imagining them. This led the doctor to say, "It's all in your head. There is no disease in your body. You are imagining the symptoms." I never saw those injunctions work effectively for a single patient.

I did turn to psychiatrists for help with some of my referral patients. Whenever I could not find a medical disease, I asked my psychiatric colleague to see the patient with me. By this time, I was doing complete medical workups on these patients as a way of being thorough and in an effort to find some disease to explain the symptoms and clinical state. I was still very much a believer in the mind-body dichotomy. When I asked the psychiatrists to see the patient, I (like others) was in effect saying, "I cannot find a disease in the body, so please find a disease of the mind for me."

The results I got from the psychiatric consultations were so varied that it is difficult to make any single generalization. I was struck by the fact that nearly every patient had some psychiatric disease label. I do not recall a single one whom the psychiatrist said was in good psychiatric health or of whom the psychiatrist said, "There is no psychiatric disease to explain this patient's symptom." Since I was referring the most complaining and symptom-loaded patients, this did not catch my full attention. It might be expected that each patient would have some psychiatric label, especially given my faith in the dichotomy of mind and body. After all, they had no disease in the body; therefore, they had to have a disease of the mind. Over the years, I began to have doubts about the near universality of psychiatric disease. At the time, however, I did not question the ubiquitous presence of psychiatric disorders.

What I did begin to question was the lack of any defined treatment based on the psychiatric label. Treatment recommendations were for "intensive psychotherapy" or "protracted group therapy." Occasionally, the note would say, "This patient lacks insight and is not amenable to psychotherapy." Even more troubling than the lack of a defined treatment was the failure of the psychiatrist to make any headway in relieving or helping the patients when they did enter therapy. In those years from 1962 to 1968, I did not see one patient with multiple symptoms in the body benefit from psychiatric interventions, however defined. Of course, patients with depression were greatly helped by the antidepressive drugs then coming into clinical practice.

The other troubling problem that came from my attempted collaboration with the psychiatrists was the poorly defined nomenclature of psychiatry. I realize now that the "science" of the mind was still very young and not well developed. In contrast to the emerging precision of endocrinology, psychiatry was still primitive. The terms most frequently used were "hysteria," "conversion symptoms," "hypochondriasis," and later "somatoform disorder." The definitions for these diagnoses were vague, and they did not direct a specific treatment.

At this point, all I knew was that psychiatry was no help with these patients with physical symptoms but no demonstrable disease. I continued to believe they must have some mental problem. I had not yet breached the mind-body dichotomy or the rule that the absence of a medical disease of the body meant the patient had a disease of the mind. I had not yet developed an operational conception of a broader model of disease.

My failure to be helpful to many of the patients with SUO and my frustrations with psychiatric failures made me even more determined to continue to explore the problems of these patients. I kept asking myself, If they do not have a treatable psychiatric disease, then what do these people have? It was the question that would eventually lead me to write this book.

# 6
# The Woman Who Believed She Was a Man

Despite my periodic contact with patients with multiple unexplained symptoms, most of my time was spent with patients with well-defined endocrine disorders. One such patient riveted my attention.

I first saw Eugene when he was under general anesthesia in the operating room of a large teaching hospital in the community. The surgeon and the consulting gynecologist had called me to come across town to the operating room to help them figure out what they had encountered in a routine operation for acute appendicitis. By this time, I had developed a reputation locally as a specialist in the field of disorders of sexual differentiation. Most of these were endocrine problems that involved the testicles, ovaries, or adrenal glands and all were congenital.

When I finally got to the operating room after stopping to mask up, put on greens, paper boots, and a cap, I found the surgeon and the gynecologist sitting on stools and leaning against the wall. They pointed to the table, where the patient was still under general anesthesia. They wanted me to look in the abdomen and give them some explanation for what they had found. Both regowned and I joined them at the operating table.

Apparently the surgeon had begun operating for acute appendicitis on what he thought was a young man. When he got into the abdominal cavity, he found not only acute appendicitis but all the internal organs of a normal female. He then called in the gynecologist, who called me.

There they were—ovaries, fallopian tubes, and a fully developed uterus. I scrubbed and gowned up so I could palpate the organs and get more direct information. I could feel the uterine cervix at the end of the uterus and below it what I thought could be the upper vaginal vault.

I asked them to undrape the patient so I could examine the external genitalia. I saw what appeared to be a perfectly normal penis. Despite all efforts, I could not find any masses that might represent testicles in the external areas of his skin. There are patients who are called "true hermaphrodites." These people have both testicles and ovaries and all sorts of combinations of internal and external genitalia—a very rare condition, but frankly, it was my first bet.

I asked the surgeon to tell me what he knew. He knew the man not only as a patient but also as an acquaintance. The patient was prominent in the northern part of the state in business and politics. Thirty-five years old, he had married his high school sweetheart and they had adopted a boy and a girl. Both the surgeon and the gynecologist had played golf with him.

I suggested they do several things. First, complete the appendectomy to reduce the chance of infection. I asked them then to biopsy what I thought were ovaries and have the pathologist call me when he had the frozen sections ready. I needed to know if there was any hint of testicular tissue present, if these were just ovaries, or both. The surgeons should then continue with a complete hysterectomy and remove all internal genital tissue. At that point, we huddled for a very confidential talk.

The situation was extremely delicate. I had a tragic experience with another adult patient, who committed suicide when some insensitive physician had told the person outright that "he" was actually a "she." I didn't want to see something like that happen again. It was not going to be easy to keep the facts quiet, but I thought it essential to protect the patient from the cruel and unneeded harm that would come if any of the findings leaked out. The three of us took a vow to cover up all the findings once we figured out what was going on. An emerging literature also confirmed the great harm and suicides that can be triggered by bluntly telling people reared in one sex that they are the opposite sex. The literature of that time indicated that forced switches in gender after the age of two years were more often harmful than helpful. (I am not discussing trans-sexuals or any conditions for which I have no experience or useful knowledge. I am referring only to patients with ambiguous external or internal genitalia.)

While the surgeons were finishing the appendectomy and the biopsy of the "ovaries," I discussed the case with the pathologist. We agreed we would label everything in ambiguous terms, such as "gonads" or "internal genitalia structures." We would avoid all use of "testicle" or "ovary" or "uterus" or anything that would specify male or female. We agreed to stick closely to the "fact" that this was a man who had some disorder with his "internal genitals" and that they had just not developed perfectly.

I then met the wife in the waiting room downstairs. She was totally unaware of the drama unfolding in the operating room. I told her everything was going along fine with the appendectomy and that her husband was in very good condition. I then told her the surgeon had uncovered the gonads and some genital tissue in the operative field. This was what I needed to discuss with her, I said, because we thought the best thing to do would be to remove these tissues because they were not functional and because they could serve only as potentials for cancer later on. I stuck as close to the facts as I could, using generic terms as much as possible, and guessing that she at least knew her husband did not have testicles that were descended. I also knew that they had adopted children. I asked her to tell me what she knew about his "undescended tes-ticles," and here I used that term on purpose.

She seemed relieved to know her husband was in no danger and proceeded to tell me in considerable detail the history of her husband's health and their life together. He had developed sexually very early, she thought around age five or six. He was shaving his face when he was eleven years old. Despite this precocious development of beard and pubic hair, he had never "dropped his testicles." That was the way she described the undescended testicles.

She had known all this while they were dating. They were very open with each other and kept no secrets. She then told me they had tried to have children for several years unsuccessfully after they married. They had even seen several doctors, who told them his testicles were undescended and that was the cause of his infertility. One physician told them his testicles would have to be removed one day if they were to prevent cancer (there was a well-known increased risk of testicular cancer in undescended testicles). Despite these contacts with physicians, he had never had a "sperm count." She then volunteered in explicit terms how wonderful their sexual life had been and continued to be. Apparently, her husband had been able to achieve full erection and penetration. Both were capable of achieving orgasm. However, to her knowledge, he had never ejaculated.

Keep in mind that this was the 1960s. Careful study of sexual development was just beginning. Chromosome counts were just becoming available, so it was no surprise that he had not had what we would now call a complete workup earlier in his life.

I had only one more set of questions for the wife. "Tell me what you know about his early growth and development. Was he a slow or fast grower? Was he short or tall for his age group growing up?" I had narrowed down the possibilities for his medical problem, and this information would pin down the last few facts I needed.

She told me he grew extremely rapidly before the first grade and continued to grow until he was around nine years old, when he stopped completely. Her husband had often commented how he went from being the tallest and largest of his class in school in his early life to being one of the shortest in his teens. It was a classic history for one of two things.

Here is what I learned from his wife with my question. The husband had developed male secondary sexual characteristics at a very early age—increase in facial hair, growth of his "penis." Most importantly in unraveling the case, he had a very rapid early growth spurt with early cessation of growth.

The wife had few questions and was relieved to know her husband was doing all right with the operation. After she agreed to have the "abnormal genital tissue removed," I headed for the pathologist's office. I had narrowed down the possible explanations to two, and the biopsy of the man's gonads would help make the final determination.

The pathologist was bent over his microscope when I walked in. Like the offices of many good pathologists, his was a mess. There were open books on every surface and wooden slide boxes stacked in between the books, journals, and papers. I could barely find a path to him among all the clutter. The place smelled like hot wax and formalin. He was mumbling to himself, unaware I had come into the room.

"What do you see?" I asked.

"Where did you get this one?" he answered, without looking up from the scope. He and I knew each other from some shared conferences at the medical school.

I told him all I wanted to know was whether it was testicle, ovary, or a combination.

"It's ovary all the way. The follicles all look early and there is some fibrosis. This is the ovary of a fertile female."

I looked into the scope and saw what he showed me with his teaching pointer from his side of the double scope. I could hear myself breathing fast around the eyepieces and sensed the urgency to arrive at a decision both accurately and quickly. The patient was lying on the table waiting for us to make up our minds. For a brief moment, I lived the life of a surgical pathologist.

I then repeated my little lecture about the crucial need to hide everything we found. The pathologist and I agreed to use generic terms. We would avoid any terms that hinted of female or uterus, including the term "hysterectomy," which was the operation I had recommended. We agreed to omit the pathology and operative report from the medical record but to keep it in a personal file in the pathologist's office under lock and key. These were the days of paternalism, and we thought nothing of withholding such information. Looking back, I still think we made the right decision.

I headed back to the operating room. The surgeon, gynecologist, and I huddled off to one side so none of the other team members would overhear us. I have always believed patients in operating rooms can "hear" at some unconscious level, and this was one time I wanted to be sure the patient had no chance of overhearing anything at any level.

Here was the way I put the case together to them. I believed this patient had congenital adrenal hyperplasia, so-called virilizing adrenal hyperplasia; this meant simply that, before he was born, the adrenals made excessive male hormones (androgens). "He" was actually a female, probably with XX sex chromosomes. His fetal androgens, coming not from testicles but from the adrenals, caused the phallus (clitoris, in this case) to fuse with the urethra and form what appeared at birth to be a normal penis. The child was born with what appeared to be undescended testicles; there was no reason to presume otherwise in that era. So he was called a little boy and raised as one.

The formation of the internal genitalia are not driven or affected by androgens but are directed by some signal from the chromosomes. Thus, they remained the normal female ovaries, fallopian tube, and uterus we saw in the abdomen.

All of this embryology and endocrinology had just been worked out in detail in animals and was only now being applied to cases in humans. There was a beauty to the embryological story that had been discovered, so sequential and understandable. And like all human systems, it could go awry—as it had in this patient.

Both the surgeon and gynecologist were listening intently.

I went on. Actually, the child would have been a perfectly normal female except for the presence of excessive androgens from a defect in the adrenal gland. The androgens after birth caused him to grow rapidly and to develop male secondary sexual characteristics at an early age (the growth of the penis and facial hair his wife told me about). The cessation of growth came from the great acceleration of bone development that comes from male hormones (androgens) and the closure of the bone-growth centers when the "bone age" reaches about sixteen years. This accelerated growth normally occurs at puberty, but in this patient's case the androgens were excessive from birth. The surgeon asked me why the patient did not menstruate or develop breasts at the age of puberty. It was a good question.

The answer is that the ovaries were suppressed by the androgens. In addition, the androgens opposed the action of estrogen at the tissue level, thus preventing the patient from menstruating through his penis. Male hormones will usually override female hormones and dominate the biologic scene, both during fetal development and later in life. In mild forms of this condition, menstruation has occurred in some cases, to the great consternation of everyone. Usually they think it is bleeding from the kidneys, and everyone is shocked to find a uterus in an otherwise normal "boy." That did not happen here because the androgen levels were probably very high and completely suppressed all estrogen effects.

I told the surgeon and the gynecologist that I ruled out a rare masculinizing/androgen-secreting tumor because the process began before birth; a tumor that secretes androgens is never congenital. I was also willing to rule out the patient's being a true hermaphrodite, since we could find no testicular tissue. But a correct biologic diagnosis was irrelevant. What we had to decide was beyond such a limited consideration. It was clear that the removal of all internal genitalia, including the ovaries, was justified.

We had now to arrive at what to say. It was clear to me that the patient was a fully functioning man, married, and responsible for two adopted children. I could think of no good and plenty of harm from laying out all the facts. It seemed to me that our responsibility was to do everything we could to assist him in remaining the best possible man he could be. This meant removing all tissue which served no male purpose and which could be a source of cancer in later life. The ovaries, tubes, uterus, and cervix all fit into this category. We agreed to call the operation an excision of "aberrant gonadal and genital tissue." We would write that in the progress notes and omit the written operative report and the pathology report from his record.

After the operation, we collected some urine and confirmed the very high levels of adrenal androgens and the diagnosis of congenital adrenal hyperplasia. (It is too complicated to go into here, but there were other aspects of his treatment that were necessary to keep him hormonally a male and deal with the adrenal hyperplasia.)

I saw the patient awake and in person only once. I really did not need to see him at all after the operation, but I think my curiosity was just too much for me. He was short, about five feet three inches, heavily bearded, and very muscular. He looked athletic and he was. His voice was quite deep. Everything about his demeanor was masculine, even a bit macho. We chatted about his golf game. I offered to answer questions. He had none, so I left after a few minutes. He later ran for public office, and I saw his picture in the papers and on television a number of times.

•  •  •

I marveled (and still do) at the wonder of being one thing at one level and believing in and behaving as something totally differently at another level. Here in one sense was indeed a "woman" (female by chromosomes, gonads, and internal genitalia) who thought "she" was a "man," so much so that it was impossible for all who knew him to tell the difference between him and any other man.

I reflected on how critical differences can be so small. There is only one hydrogen atom's difference between the molecules of estrogen and testosterone. One small hydrogen atom distinguishes all men from all women. Add a hydrogen atom to the basic molecule and you get testosterone and males. Subtract a hydrogen atom and you get estrogen and females. Is that one hydrogen atom the biochemical rib of man?

Beyond all else, the case illustrated the power of thought and belief. I didn't make the connection then, but I later related this patient to my emerging interest. If a person thinks he is sick, he is sick. If he believes he has a disease, he will behave as if he has that disease. The corollary is just as true. If a person believes he is well, then he will act as if he is well. And as in this patient, if a person thinks he is a man, he will act as if he is a man. Perception is reality. How else can we explain some people with severe disease who function so well, while others with little disease do so poorly? Each person's perception of illness is in some sense a choice that can be influenced by what the physician says and does.

I became determined to learn how to change perceptions from unhealthy ones to healthy ones.

# 7
# Mind and Body

From 1968 to 1973, I served as dean of the School of Medicine at the University of Alabama in Birmingham. My odyssey had washed me onto the shore of a strange land of parents, faculty, state legislators, fiscal officers, lawyers, and federal regulators; most of them were angry about something or wanted something. By the time I learned the language and mores of these strange people, I resigned. I had been dean for nearly five years when the average tenure was closer to two. The sirens who had called me to medical administration stopped singing their seductive songs. The calmer and more familiar waters of clinical medicine called me again.

My years in the dean's job allowed me to detach myself for a while from being a physician—in a sense, to lose my identity as a physician—but gain a sense of irony about medicine and its practice. As a state medical school, we had an obligation to consider the health of the people of the state. I began to wonder about the real causes of disease from a population basis.

At the end of my deanship, I decided to redirect my clinical interests from pure endocrinology to a broader look at illness, particularly at patients with symptoms but no medical disease. I had begun to ask myself, "If these people do not have a medical disease, then what is their problem?" To address that question, I had to do a considerable amount of retooling of my clinical skills. I had to learn much more about interviewing and listening.

During my last year as dean, I met and worked weekly with Dr. Joseph Sapira. Joe Sapira was doubly trained in psychiatry and internal medicine. He came from Pittsburgh, at the time a center and hub for faculty who were interested in the psychological aspects of illness. Sapira led me patient by patient and week by week through an understanding of the fallacy of the mind-body dichotomy. Before working with him, I had slowly begun to reject the dichotomy, but Sapira was able to reject it in a manner that also appealed to my need for scientific rigor. He was quick to point out that a stimulus or agent for disease was not limited to what could be visualized under a microscope or put in a test tube. Sounds, voices, sights, smells, colors, touches, and all the varied sensory stimuli that impinge on humans were legitimate material for scientific inquiry. Combine all of those into human communication and language and those complexes were equally legitimate material for scientific study—difficult, but amenable to direct observation and study.

I came to fully understand that the mind and the body were one—not separated, not disconnected. What affected one also affected the other. Sitting above all the molecules, tissues, organs, and mind of the human body was an integrated person. This person was connected to a family and perhaps to a spouse, and the family was connected to some social structure and society at large. All this social structure impinged on the person, and the person impinged on the social structure. There was a continuum all the way from society to the person to the organs and even down to the molecules. There were no separated pockets or islands. There certainly was no mind separated from a body.

George Engel (1977) posited such a continuum and hierarchy of interlocking subsystems in his classic paper "The Need for a New Medical Model: A Challenge for Biomedicine." He called this new model the "Bio-psycho-social Model." In 1977, when the paper was published, I read it over and over. Engel's model reinforced what Sapira had already taught me about the clinical limitations of the strictly biomolecular model. Even today, Engel's thoughts still have not received the attention they should.

It may seem strange that I am describing my transition from a belief that the mind and body were separated to one that saw no separation. I don't think I would have put it in such stark terms in the 1970s, but that is the way most physicians of that day functioned. I was no exception. Even today, some physicians still function as if the body and mind are separate and disconnected entities. This erroneous view is part of the explanation for our excessive use of procedures and technology.

In addition to having an integrated model of humans and disease, Sapira was also a superb teacher of interviewing techniques. Foremost, he was a first-order bedside clinician and would later capture much of his wisdom in his masterpiece, *The Art and Science of Bedside Diagnosis* (1999). At the beginning of mentoring me in interviewing techniques, Sapira had me see patients with him. Later he assigned me patients on my own. He had me tape-record the sessions. We then listened to the tapes together. From time to time as we listened to the tapes, he asked what I was thinking, or why I asked a specific question, or what I thought of a patient's response. He timed with a stopwatch the period between the end of a patient's answer and the beginning of my next question. At first, he noted, I waited barely two or three seconds. He taught me to make longer and longer pauses. He showed me that the longer the wait, the richer the material offered by the patient. My allowing the anxiety level to rise in the patient elicited from the patient information that would not have come in response to a direct question. I also learned to notice that the last thing a patient said as I left the room was often the most revealing and important information of the entire session. I was learning to go deeper than the superficial level of physical symptoms. I found it possible to be both observer and participant, keeping a third eye and ear on the interchange. I also was beginning to make a slight but definite change in my behavior with patients.

In addition to learning from Joe Sapira, I had the privilege of meeting and studying with the psychologist Carl Rogers in La Jolla, California. I had read Rogers's book, *On Becoming a Person* (1961). It was one of those few books of a lifetime that struck me to my core. Books like that, at least for me, always come at a special time, when there is a readiness to absorb what the author is saying. Carl Rogers left a deep and lasting impression on me through both his writings and his person. He laid out in some detail what listening was about and described the process of true listening. Some people call the process "active listening": The listener reflects back what has been heard until there is mutual agreement between listener and speaker.

Rogers had also formulated a school of psychotherapy called "client-centered therapy." This became widely known as Rogerian psychotherapy. The notion, in very brief and too abbreviated terms, held that people have the internal resources to heal their own psychological problems. Rogers believed that at the center of each person there is a core of goodness. The psychotherapist had only to facilitate that core into action by very careful listening to the person. The listening itself, to a large extent, was the therapy.

It is far beyond the scope of this book to go into more detail about what Rogers had to say. I knew one thing. I wanted to spend time with him and learn directly from him. I had been fortunate to train with his son, Dr. David Rogers, who had been chair of medicine at Vanderbilt when I was a senior resident on his service in 1959–60. Thus I had a path through David toward working with Carl Rogers.

David Rogers went on to an illustrious medical career until his early death in the 1990s. After his time as chief of medicine at Vanderbilt, where he was an active investigator of infectious diseases, he became dean of the School of Medicine at Johns Hopkins. After Hopkins, he served as the first president of the Robert Wood Johnson Foundation. There, he set the direction for the foundation and established many of its national programs. One of these, Human

Dimensions in Medicine, was championed by his father, Carl Rogers. I participated in the course and experiences of Human Dimensions in Medicine and got to know Carl himself. A widespread public belief then held that medicine had become cold and detached. Medicine needed to be humanized, and the program's intent was to introduce academic physicians to the notion that human behavior and emotions were vital considerations in clinical medicine, in medical education, and in personal development and health.

As I ended my time as dean in Birmingham, I asked for and obtained a sabbatical to regroup and further retrain my clinical skills. I also had to decide what I was going to do professionally. All I knew then was that I no longer wanted to be dean, and that I wanted to return to clinical medicine. My odyssey took me to California. I joined Carl Rogers at his Center for the Study of the Person in La Jolla in 1973. The offices of the center sat high above the seemingly endless Pacific Ocean. It was an idyllic setting. On a clear day, I could sometimes see pods of whales surface in the distance, rising from some unfathomable depth.

When I spent time with Carl, I was quite sure that he had nothing on his mind except trying to understand what I was saying and thinking. I had never experienced such full, undiluted, and riveted attention. He seemed to draw the words out of my mouth and somehow helped me to express myself more fully and more accurately. He would continue to gently rephrase what I had said until I agreed with his rephrasing. He had a remarkable listening talent, which he describes in detail in *On Becoming a Person*.

The seminars and contacts with the fellows at the Center for the Study of the Person led me to a much deeper understanding of both human communication and myself. Many of the seminars were conducted as experiential learning sessions, with the focus limited to the interactions between the people in the room. We could discuss or introduce into the conversation nothing outside the room. These "sensitivity sessions" were sometimes also called "T groups" (*t* for "training"). I found these to be intense learning sessions where feelings and emotions surfaced and forced the group to consider them. These highly personal sessions led to strong learnings about myself, my feelings, triggers for my feelings, and my relationships with others. For the first time in my life, I faced my emotions head-on. There is no way to be emotionally dishonest in such groups. I was undergoing significant and beneficial personal psychotherapy without calling it that.

In addition to the sensitivity sessions, there were case presentations of clients being seen by the fellows at the center. I rotated among the fellows and continued my daily work with Rogers. My time at the Center for the Study of the Person deepened my desire to return to clinical medicine and test my emerging ideas about medical patients, especially by examining psychological influences on medical diseases.

At the end of my sabbatical, I was ready and excited to be returning to clinical medicine and greatly relieved to be out of the dean's role. I was most fortunate to have received an offer to return to Vanderbilt to establish the Vanderbilt teaching service in medicine at Saint Thomas Hospital in Nashville and to spend a significant amount of my time exploring my new clinical directions. The timing of the offer was perfect. It was exactly what I had hoped for. I insisted that I have no income dependent on my seeing patients: I wanted to turn in all my patient-care billings, so that what I did clinically would have no bearing on my income. Grant Liddle, then chair of medicine, agreed. Vanderbilt was my intellectual home, and returning home is nearly always sweet.

My journey in one sense was bringing me back to my homeland. In another sense, my redirected clinical odyssey was just beginning. I would soon be in another strange land with a new language, feeling my way along. I have always enjoyed uncertainty.

# 8
# Sweet Thing

One of my first patients when I returned to Vanderbilt in 1973 was a teenager—"Sweet Thing," her grandmother called her. The nickname was unintentionally ironic; the girl's mother had died in her sleep with diabetes mellitus the year before. The exact proximate cause of death was unknown. All I ever heard was that the mother was thirty-six years old and that she died from the diabetes in her sleep in the front room of the house.

Sweet Thing was fifteen years old and complained of severe pain below her knees in both legs. The pain went from just below the knees to the tips of her toes. She had been diagnosed with diabetes mellitus about two years before I saw her. She had been taking NPH long-acting insulin from the time of the initial diagnosis. According to her grandmother, in whose home she lived, Sweet Thing did not take good care of herself, had frequent insulin reactions, and did not follow her diet or test her urine for glucose the way she should.

(In those days, only urine sugar was tested at home. Serial blood glucose ambulatory monitoring had not been invented. In fact, most physicians did not yet believe that tight control of blood glucose made any long-term difference. The national clinical trial of tight control versus usual control of blood glucose was still in the future.)

After my initial workup, which was normal, I began to see

Sweet Thing at weekly intervals until I could get a better understanding of what was going on, in particular with the leg pains. Any
kind of neurological complication would be unusual after only two
years of juvenile diabetes (that was what we called type 1 diabetes in those days). My neurological examination was normal and
showed no evidence for the peripheral neuropathy her family physician had said she had. I then wrote for her records from the family
physician.

During the first week of follow-up she had an insulin reaction
almost daily. Her fasting blood sugar on the day I saw her was 60
mg/dL. I suggested she lower the dose of insulin from twenty units
in the morning to fifteen units daily. The next week she told me she
had continued to have insulin reactions. I still did not have the family physician's records and asked the grandmother to call and prod
the physician to send them. Again I lowered the insulin dose. I continued to see Sweet Thing weekly, and each time I lowered the dose
of insulin. The insulin reactions continued, so I suggested she stop
the insulin and carefully follow her urine sugars. The grandmother
was to call me if anything untoward occurred, particularly if she
began to spill sugar heavily in the urine.

I was having a difficult time trying to figure out what was going on. Was this some unusual and delayed remission of the disease? Did she have some other disease that was ameliorating the
diabetes? Did she even have diabetes in the first place? I had seen
patients who had false diagnoses of diabetes mellitus, but I had not
seen one this young or anyone who had been given insulin for a
false diagnosis of the disease. This case was unusual, whatever the
answer would turn out to be.

I saw Sweet Thing twice a week during the stoppage of insulin. She suffered no further hypoglycemic reactions while she was
off the insulin. That would be expected. What was remarkable was
that her blood sugars remained normal even up to three weeks after I stopped her insulin. Finally, the records came from the family
doctor.

When the family doctor first saw Sweet Thing two years before, she told him she had tested her own urine with her mother's urine-testing kit and found sugar in her urine. The physician ordered a five-hour glucose-tolerance test. The test called for a 100-gram oral glucose load. Blood sugars were measured every half-hour for the first two hours, then every hour. The value rose to about 150 mg/dL at one hour and fell back to normal by one-and-a-half hours. At one hour, she showed a positive test for sugar in the urine, which stayed positive for another hour and then became negative. It was a normal glucose-tolerance-test result. Usually, glucose spills into the urine when the blood glucose is greater than 180mg/dL. Sweet Thing spilled glucose at a level of 150mg/dL. She thus had renal glycosuria, a benign condition, not diabetes mellitus.

Biased by the strong family history of diabetes mellitus, the physician had made an erroneous diagnosis of diabetes based solely on the positive urine sugar. He started her immediately on insulin. How she had tolerated the insulin for two years without more obvious brain damage is still a puzzle.

The false diagnosis of diabetes in Sweet Thing had triggered several unfortunate behaviors in her family. First, her grandmother, still grieving the death of her daughter and now worried about her granddaughter, made a firm resolve to see to it that her granddaughter took better care of herself. Sweet Thing's mother had severe diabetes with renal failure and near blindness before she died. To make sure Sweet Thing followed the diabetic diet and took her insulin, the grandmother had insisted on taking the girl to the local city hospital clinic to see all the amputated diabetic patients who sat around the waiting room in wheelchairs. She told Sweet Thing that she would end up like the people she saw if she did not follow the diet and take the insulin. The girl told me that the leg pains came on after that visit. However, she did not seem to make the connection in any causative way.

The second and even more serious consequence of the diagnosis was the nearly complete social withdrawal that her brothers and sisters forced on Sweet Thing after their mother died in her sleep. They made her sleep alone in the very room where their mother had died. All of them were already afraid to sleep in that room. Now they were afraid to sleep in the same room with their sister, for fear she too would die in her sleep. She said that one of her brothers told her, "I ain't gonna sleep in no room with somebody who's gonna die in the night." They moved to the rooms at the back of the large house, leaving Sweet Thing to sleep alone in the vacated front room. The girl stayed awake late into the nights wondering if she would die and when it might happen. She also lived in fear of losing her legs and had no one to turn to, since all but her grandmother had turned away from her.

Her grandmother refused to believe me when I told the family that Sweet Thing did not have diabetes. They insisted that the family doctor was correct, and that I was making a mistake to stop the insulin. How did I explain the sugar in the urine if she did not have diabetes? I asked for a repeat of the glucose-tolerance test, thinking that a normal test the second time would persuade them to believe me. The family agreed. The test was normal with the blood sugar levels; however, Sweet Thing again spilled glucose in the urine at barely elevated blood glucose levels—again documenting the low renal threshold for glucose. When I went over the results, the family still refused to believe the girl did not have diabetes.

The grandmother said, "What you mean she ain't got sugar diabetes? She got sugar in her urine just like her momma had."

I wrote the family doctor a full report, giving my diagnosis of renal glycosuria, the story of the insulin withdrawal, and the persistence of normal blood sugars even in the absence of administered insulin. I never saw the grandmother or the patient again. Through a relative of the girl that worked in the hospital, I learned a few months later that the family doctor had put the girl back on insulin and that the family still refused to sleep in the same room with her.

I failed to convince either Sweet Thing or her grandmother of the error of the diagnosis of diabetes. Both seemed determined to hold onto it despite all my efforts. Their position was reinforced by the family doctor, in whom they had complete trust. I had also failed to convince him of the error.

Head-on, I had witnessed the power of strongly held beliefs. Perception is indeed reality, even if the "facts" are in error. The grandmother, Sweet Thing, and the family doctor believed Sweet Thing had diabetes. I had experienced the failure of facts and logic when they came up against the raw power of belief.

• • •

Looking back from the vantage point of more than twenty-five years later, I can see my error in insisting on removing the label of diabetes. My insistence had only pushed the family further into lack of trust. What we called the condition was unimportant, so long as we did not let the label dictate harmful treatment or procedures. I would learn this, but only in later patients. I wish now I had just removed the insulin and continued to follow the girl along. In time, we might have convinced Sweet Thing and her grandmother that she was not on the same dreadful course as her dead mother. I still had a lot to learn about persuasion.

I also was beginning to sense the need for physicians to examine their own beliefs and separate those that are important for the patient from those that are important to themselves. My extreme need at the time to use accurate medical terminology overrode what might have been best for the care of this frightened girl and her family.

Up until this point, I had assumed that assigning a nonexistent disease name to a patient was just sloppy medicine, a poor method for dealing with symptomatic patients. I considered it a lazy way out. It did not fit my test for eloquence in the diagnostic process.

I now see the error of overdiagnosing a nonexistent disease as powerful evidence for why we need to abandon the biomolecular model for clinical medicine. It was not until I reflected on Sweet

Thing and my own errors in her management that I came to this broader view of the origins of the error of nondisease. The error is not sloppy medicine. It is an error demanded by a paradigm that restricts diseases to either the body or the mind. This paradigm relegates human beings to an isolated island of brain, other organs, tissues, cells, and molecules disconnected from the narrative of life.

# 9
# New Clinical Interventions

It became apparent to me that I needed to set some definitions around what I was doing clinically. Since returning to Vanderbilt and Saint Thomas, I had begun to see a large number of referred patients. Word got around that I was interested in seeing patients who had symptoms of disease but no objective evidence of disease. Many of these were labeled "difficult" or "problem" patients. Some referring physicians called them by pejorative terms—"crock" or "turkey" or "shad." The physicians were, in most cases, very glad to send such patients to me for continued care. They seemed happy to have the patients out of their practice.

I arrived at a standardized approach for patients with symptoms of unknown origin (SUO) referred to me for management or for consultations. I defined SUO as symptoms of more than a month's duration for which there was no readily apparent medical disease to explain them. The patient may or may not already carry a diagnosis of a disease. I did not use this standardized approach when the medical diagnosis and thus the therapy were obvious early in the visit or consultation. For example, I did not use this approach with most patients I saw who had classic endocrine diseases (hyperthyroidism, hypothyroidism, Cushing's syndrome, and other well-defined endocrine excesses or deficiencies).

Here is the approach I set out to use:

1.  I would not make a diagnosis unless I had convincing evidence for the presence of the disease.
2.  I would do a comprehensive medical workup on each patient, focusing on the symptoms when appropriate.
3.  I would use Joseph Sapira's injunction frequently: "I do not know what you have . . . *yet.*"
4.  I would continue to tell the patient about those diseases that I knew with near certainty were *not* present.
5.  I would not attempt to make a psychiatric diagnosis except for depression, which I saw as a treatable and diagnosable disease.
6.  I would put equal value on physical, psychological, or social information offered by the patient. I did not care if the underlying causes were psychological, social, physical, or all three. My goal was to uncover and address the source of the patient's distress.
7.  I would ask the patient to keep a daily symptom diary. The timing of entries depended on the frequency of the symptom—some entries were to be made hourly, some every four hours, some twice a day, and some daily. The symptoms were graded zero to ten on each entry. I used a very severe definition of ten: that level of unpleasantness (pain, intensity) for which you might seriously consider suicide. Zero was an absence of the symptom.

    The other data to be entered in the diary depended on the location and nature of the symptom. For example, if the symptom was in the GI (gastrointestinal) tract, I had patients list the foods eaten; if in the respiratory system, I had them make observations on what they were breathing or smelled. I had nearly all patients pay special attention to the people they encountered in each recording period.

(My goal here was to have the patient begin to draw correlations between the symptom and the world around them. I was looking for a variation or "wobble" of the symptom and then examining what preceded the "wobble.")

8.  When and if the patient discovered some substance, event, or person that seemed to correlate with or precede the symptom, I would suggest that he or she eliminate the substance or confront the situation and see what happened to the symptom.

9.  If the patient could not identify a correlation between the symptom and any stimulus in his or her life, I would use the following questions, which became some of my favorites: "Is there something in your life that you should stop doing? Or is there something in your life that you are not doing that you should be doing?" (Notice how unspecified the language is. I will have more to say about the extraordinary power of unspecified language in later chapters.)

10. I would have the patient continue the diary process until the symptoms went away or became manageable, or we established a cause or medical disease to explain them. In some cases, the process failed or the patient refused to adhere to the approach or left to see another physician.

There were several reasons for my decision to avoid psychiatric labels (number 5 on the list). Most important, perhaps, no treatment existed for the illnesses described by most of the psychiatric labels that might fit these patients. Also, such terms as "hypochondriasis," "hysteria," or "somatizing disorder" would become labels that would interfere with my systematic approach. In addition, in the past I had referred such patients to psychiatrists with no benefit.

Finally, I had engaged Dr. Harry Abram, head of Liaison Psychiatry at Vanderbilt, to serve as my mentor so that I would have psychiatric backup if I got in over my head. Dr. Abram and I met on a regular basis to review the case histories until his sudden and untimely death in 1977.*

It was and still is my strong belief that many of these patients can be handled only by physicians well trained in internal medicine. (Sharing these experiences with such physicians is one of my motives for writing this book.) At the outset, there is no way to know if a psychological or physical cause or a combination of the two will be found to explain the symptom. Premature jumps to psychiatric labels are not appropriate and create avoidable problems. Some of these patients ping-pong back and forth between a medical doctor and a psychiatrist. The medical doctor insists the problem is psychiatric. The psychiatrist, sometimes frightened by the physical symptoms, refers the patient back to the medical doctor. The patient goes back and forth and gets no real help.

Over the next several years, I saw an increasing number of patients with SUOs. (See Chapter 11 for a detailed analysis of a subset of these patients.) After I did further study, I found that the patients I saw fell into one of the following categories:

1.  The patient had a hidden or obscure medical disease that explained the symptoms.
2.  The patient had an identifiable psychosocial stress that produced the symptoms.
3.  The patient was unknowingly ingesting, inhaling, or contacting a substance that produced the symptoms.
4.  The patient had a self-induced disease that produced the symptoms or findings.
5.  The patient denied the existence or even the possibility of any biopsychosocial stress as a cause of the symptoms.

---

*I am fortunate to have known and worked with Harry Abram. Much of the substance of this book comes from his wisdom.

(These patients remained symptomatic; see Group IV in Chapter 11.)

The patient stories in the chapters that follow illustrate some of these causes for SUO. In addition, the stories show the progressive complexity of my interventions and my increasing attention to methods of communication with the patients. In some of the stories, I begin to apply the same interventions and methods of communication to patients with known medical diseases but whose symptoms were difficult to control. With those patients, I begin to bridge a psychological approach with medical management.

# 10
# Florence's Symptoms

Florence was a plain woman. Although she had never been in a psychiatric hospital, her hair was cut like most back-ward psychiatric patients—straight bob with bangs, as you might imagine some rushed attendant would cut it. Her hair was uncombed, tangled, and dirty. She wore a colorless smock, an oversized sweater, no stockings, and brown oxfords with low sturdy heels. She looked down at the floor as she talked. My first impression was of a very disturbed woman who had just about given up on life.

Florence and Sweet Thing (Chapter 8) were my first patients on my new venture into clinical medicine when I returned to Vanderbilt on the full-time faculty to run the medical teaching program at Saint Thomas Hospital. With plenty of patient-care time and no income dependence, I could test my new ideas and approaches to patients. I had the best of all clinical worlds.

I asked Florence why she had come to see me, and her response was that she hoped I could find out what was wrong with her. To say she was overdoctored is an understatement. She was then seeing at least seven specialists, including a psychiatrist. She had seen innumerable others in the preceding years. In my initial history, which took over an hour, she gave a bewildering array of complaints, more than thirty symptoms that covered nearly all areas of the body. I told her that I did not know what she had *yet*, but that I would give her my best effort to find out. I asked that she have each of the specialists write me a letter and send me a copy of his or her records. I drafted a letter for her and had her sign the usual release form to accompany it. The physical examination would have to wait for the next visit—an omission that always evoked some guilt, a residual of my compulsive training to do both workup and exam on the first visit.

After Florence left, I reflected on her situation. It was clear she was going to be an extraordinarily difficult patient. Despite her withdrawn appearance, there was a defiant manner about her. She seemed to take some pleasure in telling me how she had tried everything the various specialists had suggested, yet all had failed to help her. She found fault with every doctor. Nobody could find out what was wrong with her, and no one had helped her. She had been on all sorts of medications. She had also undergone a long list of diagnostic procedures and surgical operations. She spent some time telling me in detail how each treatment or operation had either not helped or made her worse.

My initial plan was simple. I would get all the test results, review them, and try to find a disease that had not yet been considered. It was a strategy I had found useful for patients who presented difficult problems. The question in this setting is, "What diseases would escape detection from this battery of tests?" It is the strategy one must use in the tough referral cases. This approach of looking for the missed disease is also the correct strategy in the clinicopathological conferences (CPCs) so popular in medical schools. Having test results at the same time you are unraveling a difficult patient's symptoms is one of the great advantages of being a referral specialist. (It is a completely different clinical approach from seeing a new patient for the first time.) "What did they miss?" is the question on referred patients. One eventually develops a list of favorite missed diagnoses.

The other part of my initial plan was to stick to discussing Florence's symptoms and not digress. I was following Carl Rogers's admonition to try to be wherever the patient is—"entering the world of the patient," is the way he put it. I would play the role of medical doctor to the nth degree. Time was about the only thing on my side. As I found out over the next several weeks, I would have to use it to its full power.

During the next few visits, which I had set at weekly intervals for one hour each, I completed my physical examination—which was entirely normal—reviewed the records from the specialists, and finished recording the list of symptoms Florence described. At this point, I had no idea what she had. It was no wonder that she was seeing so many specialists. And it was no surprise that she already had several diagnoses from them.

The first and most terrifying diagnosis was what the ophthalmologist had described as an "impending detaching retina." Never having heard of such a diagnosis, I called him and discussed the case. He retracted the diagnosis. I asked why he had made the diagnosis in the first place. He answered that Florence insisted on some medical term for her symptom of floaters in her field of vision. He had told her that sometimes patients saw those when they were about to have a detached retina. It took several weeks for Florence to get that off her mind or at least to stop talking about it.

The other diagnoses she had been told about included a urinary bladder–neck obstruction, a rectal fissure, migraine headaches, low thyroid function, "weak lungs," and colitis. I could confirm none of these. She had been told that she needed to have an upper GI endoscopy, a liver biopsy, and possibly a kidney biopsy. The urologist wanted to repair the urinary bladder obstruction. She also had been told that her uterus was tilted backward and needed to be either removed or suspended (a useless but popular operation of that time).

After some considerable thought, I arrived at my first rule in dealing with Florence if I were to continue seeing her. I asked that she stop seeing all other physicians for a period of two months. Of course, she was free to see them, but if she did, I would terminate my relationship as her physician. My thinking was this: If she continued to see specialists, then about all I could do would be to get in the middle and try to interpret or second-guess what she said they had said. I had already found that what she said the specialists said and what the specialists said they said were two very different things. It was going to be a big enough job to get all Florence's symptoms identified and contained without the added problem of going over what some other physician had said. I knew it was a risky bargain to suggest, but the challenge of this woman with more than thirty symptoms combined with my strong interest in such patients was too much to resist. I saw her as a research subject, and in fact I told her exactly that. I had no idea what I had gotten myself into until her husband and mother arrived unscheduled in my office a day after I laid out the rule about seeing no other physicians.

The first thing the mother said was, "I am Florence's mother. I am a paranoid schizophrenic and she is too. This is her husband, whom I despise. What do you mean by telling Florence she cannot see another doctor?"

Before I could respond, she continued with a long, rambling exposition on her first husband, his mother, his worthlessness, the divorce, her second marriage, Florence's birth, and the disappearance of the second husband, and then a jumbled account of her many stays in psychiatric hospitals and the details of how Florence was following in her footsteps. With no conclusion to her long discursion, she left, almost in midsentence. I stood at the door not knowing what to say or do.

Florence's husband was typical of many young men of the early 1970s—a full beard, a pony tail, a huge black hat that he never removed, sandals with no socks. He wore a green uniform from some quasi-military outfit I could not identify. He could have passed as a Cuban revolutionary. He did not say a word until Florence's mother left.

He then said, in a most mellow and melodious stoned voice, "She really is a paranoid schizophrenic, but I don't think Florence is. You did right to make her stop seeing all those doctors. I'll see to it that she won't do you harm. Part of Florence's problem has got to be that mother of hers."

He talked for several minutes about Florence and her mother and how each time Florence started to improve, her mother stepped in and set everything back. He told me a little about himself. He was working on a loading dock but had plans to go to graduate or law school.

On my next visit with Florence, I restated my rule about not seeing other specialists. She agreed, and we were off on what turned out to be almost a year of weekly visits.

I had finished my calls to all the specialists she had been seeing. The urologist who thought she had a bladder-neck obstruction that needed surgical repair had already dilated her bladder neck several times with a metal sound, a common practice among some urologists, especially with women who complained of burning on urination, prominent among Florence's symptoms. The urologist was the only physician who objected to my plan and said so. I told him I would keep Florence off his back. He hung up on me. None of the other specialists liked Florence and openly told me they hated to see her coming. I asked each one to refer her back to me if she showed up without a letter from me. They all also agreed to hold off any new procedures for the two-month period, even if she did show up in their offices.

I never saw Florence's mother again, so she did not follow through on her threats. The husband came from time to time with Florence, but I talked to him only a few times after our initial visit.

All of this arranging took a lot of time in between visits, but to gain some understanding, I was determined to follow at least one patient who had a large number of symptoms until I had exhausted all efforts. Most patients with multiple symptoms jump from doctor to doctor, which gave me more motivation to follow Florence for as long as possible. The profession as a whole detested patients with many symptoms and avoided them whenever possible or dealt with them as though the organ of their specialty could be separately considered. This explains the frequency with which these patients were subjected to surgical or invasive diagnostic procedures. I have often wondered how much of the national health-care bill goes for patients like Florence and the unnecessary procedures they get.

Psychiatric nomenclature was no help to me, especially since it listed all such conditions as untreatable. Possible psychiatric terms included "hysteria" or "hypochondriasis" or "somatizing disorder" or even "malingering." Since I was omitting no definitive psychiatric therapy, and since Florence had already seen a number of psychiatrists, I decided to follow her along on my own. I really did not have a diagnosis. She had failed to respond to a large number of antidepressants. I decided that I would open my mind as much as possible and try to listen to what Florence might be saying with her symptoms. I had no clear formulation, except that I would avoid all labels for her until I was certain of my diagnosis. I would stay on the alert for any disease that might respond to medicines or surgery; I did not want to miss a treatable disease. I had decided that if I missed a disease for which there was no treatment, it would not really matter.

I would listen as carefully as possible and do testing only if I seriously suspected some disease that had not been checked before. I would rule out any likely disease that her symptoms would support (the reports from the specialists ruled out almost all such diseases I could think of). I did test for a few rare metabolic diseases that can cause diffuse and sometimes bizarre symptoms. These excluded, I proceeded to dissect her symptoms to the limit of my ability to ask questions. I was determined to define the precise nature of what she was feeling. I stuck with Carl Rogers's injunction: "Enter into the person's world."

The list of symptoms by the end of the sixth week of visits included:

Headaches
Double vision

Itching ear canals
Itching tongue
Deep pain in her throat
Shortness of breath
A dull chest pain
Fullness after eating
Pain with menses
Burning on urination
Difficulty urinating
Painful bowel movements
Constipation
Difficulty swallowing
Pain on swallowing
Aching lower legs, arms, thighs, and shoulders
Periodic nausea
Dark urine
Painful intercourse
Irregular menses
Crawling sensations under the skin of her face
Intolerance to several foods
Dizzy spells
Spots in her field of vision
Abdominal swelling
Swelling of her hands and feet
Red blotches on her neck
Hair falling out
Weak spells but no loss of consciousness
A feeling of impending doom
Sensations of being hot and cold
Tingling sensations in her legs
Decreases in visual acuity that would come and go
Episodes of severe abdominal pains
Loss of energy and tired feelings
Feeling sick all over

I listed all these on a paper and had her sign it. I went over and over the list to make certain that she had mentioned every conceivable symptom she was having. I asked her to get her husband to sign the list, so that he had his chance to add any symptom she had not told me about. I told her that in future visits we would simply not deal with any symptom that was not on the list. I was not going to have her keep adding symptoms as we went along. She agreed to this and spent some time going over her symptoms until she had them all listed. I was trying to pin her down, a difficult thing to do because she jumped from one subject or symptom to another. My idea with the list was to get her to come to some finality about something, even if it had to be a mere list of her symptoms.

At each visit, I focused on only one symptom. I hammered it into the ground. I asked what time of day it was worse, when it was better, what made it better, what made it worse, did it move around, and if so, how and in what direction. I sometimes had her draw the course of movement of the symptom on her body. I kept getting her to focus on what outside her influenced the symptom. Did something she ate or drank influence it? Were the symptoms related to people, or places, or thoughts, or moods, or day of the week, or night or day, or travel, or the smell of anything, or the sight of anything, or the sound of something specific? I developed an endless list of questions, which I methodically applied to each of her symptoms. I wanted to know how frequently she had each one, the maximum number in a day, the longest symptom-free interval. I went down the list of symptoms one by one. I never asked her how she felt or how she was getting along in a more general way. I was being a diagnostician. I was either going to make a diagnosis or wear her out in the process. I would also continue to follow the guide of Carl Rogers and be in the world of Florence. If symptoms were where she was, I would stay there with her.

She told me early that she was absolutely convinced that she had a very rare disease that was beyond medical science. I went with that notion to an absurd degree. I never gave up. I was going to find out what was wrong with her. I also kept telling her, "I do not know what is wrong with you . . . *yet.*" I never said, "I do not know what is wrong with you" without adding, with extra emphasis, the word "yet."

I never told her that "nothing was wrong" with her. The use of that phrase was and still is a popular way of dealing with patients with many symptoms. I never saw it produce anything but anger. I always thought it insulting to tell someone so miserable with so many symptoms that "nothing is wrong." If I were in the shoes of someone with many symptoms, I would think it the height of stupidity for anyone to tell me that nothing was wrong. On its surface, the statement is absurd. The statement just makes no sense. Despite the compelling logic against its use, it continues to be a popular phrase for trying to deal with these very difficult patients.

I also resisted the common course of telling such a patient that the problem was "all in your head." As with the attempt to persuade someone that nothing is wrong, I found it demeaning to tell a person racked with symptoms that it was all in his or her head. I never heard of this statement profiting anyone. I cannot imagine a patient saying, "Oh, really? It's just a matter of all those symptoms being in my head. You mean, if I just quit imagining those symptoms, they will just go away? Oh, thank you, Doctor, for such insight and help." I resisted using either phrase with Florence.

The foremost reason was that I truly did not know what patients like Florence suffered from. That lack of knowledge was what stirred my interest in her. In fact, I began to believe that each such patient suffered from something very different from the other, that there was no one disease or even a group of diseases responsible. I came to believe that each patient suffered idiosyncratically of his or her own peculiar difficulty. How could I with any accuracy say that there was nothing wrong, or that it was just something in their head? I did not know what they had and until I did, I would tell them I did not know . . . *yet.*

There were at least two other prevailing strategies for dealing with patients with many symptoms. The first, and the most dangerous, was to make a diagnostic error and assign a false diagnosis to the patient. You may recall my experiences with Dr. Drayton Doherty in Selma. This error had already occurred on several occasions and with several physicians in Florence's case. The removal of these false diagnoses took a lot of time. The diagnoses had already led to unnecessary procedures and operations. Florence had been lucky to escape complications or drug side effects. Not every such patient was as fortunate. There are very few tragedies as serious as those that occur when an operation a patient did not need in the first place does permanent harm: Thus my obsession with not assigning a diagnosis I could not prove.

The other common way of dealing with these patients was to make up an innocuous diagnosis and assign it to them. There still are a lot of these assigned diagnoses. Each has a counterpart disease that is real but difficult to substantiate, or not too serious, or not life threatening, or trivial even when proven. Many are chronic. Most do not have a clean lab test or procedure to prove their existence or absence. I do not mean to demean these conditions, but they are so often assigned that they have come to be almost meaningless for many physicians. The assignable diagnoses I am thinking about are colitis, spastic colon, dropped kidney, hiatus hernia, sinus (without specifying "itis" or any other describer), bronchitis, migraines, allergies of all sorts (especially allergies to foods), gastritis, or gastroenteritis. Bladder-neck tightness is a popular one, especially for women. There are dozens of these diagnoses. The point in using them is that the patient now has "something." The common theory is that it is best to give the patient a label, even if it stretches the truth a bit to do so. It is fair to say that this is the most common method for dealing with a patient with many ill-defined symptoms. I rejected this approach also. It somehow lacked diagnostic eloquence—and, too, it was dishonest.

What I was attempting with Florence was to abandon all these common approaches, stay completely honest, and see where it led.

I would certainly not tell her it was "all in her head" or that "there was nothing wrong." I did not believe either was accurate or helpful. I would try to avoid making a diagnostic error and recommending an operation or drugs for some disease I overdiagnosed. I would also not make up some diagnosis just to satisfy my need for one or to give Florence a sense of certainty about her symptoms when no certainty existed. I would stay as close to dead-level honesty as I possibly could. I would experience where this approach led. And there was one final thing I would try: I would tell Florence in great detail what I knew she did *not* have.

I now had a very long list of diseases I knew she did not have, and in some sessions, I would read the list very slowly to her. I would say, "I now know you do not have tuberculosis or histoplasmosis or any of the deep fungal infections. You do not have adrenal insufficiency, or adrenal hyperfunction or pituitary hypo- or hyperfunction. You do not have low thyroid function or high thyroid function. You do not have mitral valve disease or pulmonary valve disease or aortic valve disease." I would go on and on in boring detail, dragging out my list of absent diseases.

Florence was formally well educated and an intellectual. Her undergraduate major was in German. She had a master's in English literature and she was two years into her Ph.D. degree in history. She read constantly and had focused much of her recent reading on the medical literature, which she had access to through the graduate library. She was a constant challenge, bringing me articles and references about different diagnostic possibilities. Each time, I methodically went through why she did not have the latest disease she had found in the literature. In some cases, I actually ordered the test that would confirm or refute the suggested disease. Many of them were tropical diseases or infestations unknown in the United States. On a number of occasions, I tested her stool for worms of various sorts, even though I thought it highly unlikely that she had any of them or that they could be causing the symptoms she had. I learned a lot of medicine from Florence and thanked her for her

efforts. I kept telling her that I did not know what she had . . . *yet.*
All I could do was keep trying to take the most complete history I
could on her agreed-upon list of symptoms.

Then one day as I was going down the list of diseases I knew
she did not have, she started to laugh. I had laughed frequently
about some of her symptoms, but this was the first time I had heard
her laugh. She laughed and laughed until her eyes were watering.
I waited. After she collected herself, she said, "Okay, this is getting
ridiculous. It's ludicrous, that's what it is. It's ridiculous."

"Ridiculous? What's ridiculous?" I asked.

"This whole thing. This whole silly thing." Then she looked very
puzzled and sat there saying nothing, staring out the window.

I must have waited ten minutes. I could hear Sapira in my
mind's ear. "Hold out . . . hold out . . . use pauses; let the patient
speak first whenever possible." It was like holding my breath too
long under water. I wanted to say something. I wanted to ask her
ten thousand questions about what she was thinking and how she
had arrived at the idea of being ridiculous.

Then she said, with some hesitation, "I need to think. I'll see
you next time," and she left. For the first time, she was calm and deliberate. Her face looked completely relaxed with none of the lines
on her forehead. She looked like a young girl.

This occurred at the end of the ninth month. The next time she
came in, she looked very different from any time before. She was
transformed. She wore her hair in a small ponytail. Her dress was
new and colorful. She had on makeup, and she was full of talk and
movement. She leaned forward as she spoke. "I will be completely
honest with you. I have believed all along that I had only one disease. I was embarrassed to tell you what I really thought I had. I still
am, but I must tell you now because I think it is treatable." She had
latched onto my insistence on emphasizing treatable diseases as we
looked for a diagnosis.

"What do you think you have?" I asked. I had asked her that
question a dozen or more times in the past. This time, I was al-

most breathless with excitement. It was the first visit she had not launched into her litany of symptoms and the details about them she had observed in the interval.

"I think I have lice under the skin of my body, and I know they are eating my hair follicles." She blushed and looked embarrassed.

I asked her what test she thought I should do to prove the diagnosis right or wrong.

She went on to tell me that she wanted me to biopsy her skin and find the lice. I thought for several moments. I sensed we were at a critical point. I did not like the idea of doing a biopsy of her skin, especially of her face, and certainly not for such a far-fetched notion. I did not want to lose her at this point. I told her that she would most likely reject the report if the biopsy was negative and say that the lice had moved to another site just before the biopsy. Biopsies, I thought, would lead to some sort of crazy game of doing one biopsy after another. She would never be satisfied that we had done the correct site. Therefore I rejected the notion and refused to request a biopsy.

"What else might convince you that lice infestation was the one and only disease that you have or would convince you that you do not have lice? What can I do that would do that for you?" I asked, still having no idea where this would lead. I did acknowledge to myself and in the way I phrased my response that we had arrived at a point of only one disease. I ignored for the moment the fact that medical science did not recognize lice under the skin as even possible.

She thought for several minutes and said, "Treat me for lice and I will be satisfied."

I said I would have to think about that a long time; that I had an inviolate rule that I never treated for a disease unless I had firm evidence that the disease was present; that in fact I thought it was unethical to treat people for diseases that were not present. I ended the visit early and told Florence I would consider her request.

After much thinking and soul searching, I came to a decision.

Before Florence's next visit, I had the pharmacist prepare a very dilute solution of Qwell lotion (the current highly effective treatment for body lice and one Florence had already looked up in the books). On the next visit, I wrote her the one and only prescription I had written for her in the nine months I had been seeing her. I suggested she apply the lotion to her whole body twice daily for ten days. I did not want her to miss a spot, so I spent some time telling her exactly how she should apply the liquid. I put myself into whatever mental gear I thought might increase the potency of the placebo, if a placebo was going to work here.

She smiled as I handed the prescription to her, and then she said, "But you do know, don't you, that you must treat again in two weeks to kill the eggs that hatch after the first treatment?"

I agreed to a second course, and she left. I did not make another appointment with her for a full month, the longest interval since I had been seeing her. I had very mixed feelings about having treated her with a drug for a disease I knew with some certainty did not exist. Yet I sensed it was the correct thing to do for Florence. And then I recalled old Dr. Doherty and Vanders from my earlier days. If Dr. Doherty could save a dying man with a lizard and some apomorphine, then who was I to withhold a dilute solution of Qwell?

Florence returned with her husband. Both were all smiles. She looked like an entirely different person—confident and very outgoing. She often deferred to her husband, who thanked me again and again.

Both talked of their future. He was going to go to graduate school too, in geology, I believe. She would finish her Ph.D. in history and had a job lined up with the university library research department.

We did not talk of any symptom nor did I ask Florence how she felt.

•  •  •

Over the last twenty years, I have heard from Florence from time to time. A couple of years after her last visit, she had to come into the hospital for a kidney infection, which she actually had. I was almost certain it would trigger some relapse or a return of all her symptoms. None of that happened. She got treated and left in a few days. None of the symptoms recurred. When I last talked to her on the phone a few years ago, she had not seen a physician in many years. She said she was doing fine.

I never knew what she had or what diagnosis she might be assigned. I had no idea how what I did helped or even if what I did had anything at all to do with her getting well. At times, I think I just followed someone while she went through the extraordinary course of some weird disease. At other times, I think she might have been called schizophrenic—and then I think not. I am sure many who read this will think I missed a depression with somatization. I don't think so. Besides, she had been on high-dose antidepressants and under the care of a psychiatrist with no improvement. She lacked so many of the symptoms of depression, foremost being that she never felt depressed. All I did was listen and listen and finally give her a placebo.

I thought I was following her in the world in which she found herself, namely, a world filled with physical symptoms. She was the first patient with whom all I really did was listen and talk. If such a result could happen with someone as complex as Florence, it could also happen with a lot of other patients. The experience encouraged me to continue my exploration of patients who had symptoms but no definable medical disease.

# 11
# Symptoms Without Disease

In 1976, I decided to analyze as a group the patients I had seen with symptoms of unknown origin. By then my belief that there is not a disease behind every symptom was absolute. For some patients there is no diagnosis. There is just a series of connected thoughts, actions, conflicts, and stress. The body responds with symptoms. Any misplaced diagnosis will prevent discovery of the underlying causes. When I was able to find a medical disease to explain the symptoms of a patient in this group, I excluded that patient from further analysis. These exluded patients had a variety of diseases, including mild hyperthyroidism, mild Cushing's syndrome, hypopituitarism, and porphyria cutanea tarda, a rare disorder of hemoglobin biosynthesis.

From 1973 to 1976, I saw 150 patients in whom I failed to find a medical disease to explain the symptoms. Seventy-two of these patients had coexisting and defined medical diseases; however, none of the diseases could reasonably explain the symptoms the patients complained of. Nevertheless, I excluded these patients from further detailed analysis. Examples of those I excluded were patients with hypertension, simple goiters, gallstones, hemorrhoids, varicose veins, and similar diagnoses. Although these patients had SUOs, I wanted a pure sample of people for whom there was no demonstrable disease after a thorough medical workup. Using microbiology as a metaphor, I wanted a pure culture: patients with symptoms but with no known medical diseases.

I have struggled with appropriate nomenclature for many years to avoid perpetuating the mind-body dichotomy. I do not want to make a distinction between a disease of psychological origin and one whose origin is a physically definable agent or substance. I don't want to use the terms "organic" and "functional." "Organic" implies that diseases of the body are organic or real; "functional" implies that diseases of psychological origin are not real. Here, I will use the terms "medical disease" or "objectively definable disease" or "diagnosable disease" interchangeably.

For my analysis, I excluded patients with any disease with objective findings for which there is a code in the *International Classification of Diseases* manual. I also excluded from the analysis patients with depression, although I did not exclude any of the somatizing disorders. "Somatizing disorder" is a psychiatric label for any condition in which people complain of physical symptoms but have no medical disease. I prefer the term "SUO," since it has *no* implications, psychiatric or otherwise. I also did not exclude patients with errors of refraction or caries of the teeth.

## Grouping the Patients

I was left with seventy-eight patients who had symptoms but no diagnosable or coexisting medical disease to explain the symptom. A colleague (and a wag) who was puzzled by my interest said I had a "pure culture of clinical nothingness." His comment, intended to be humorous, reflected a common attitude about these unfortunate patients: "If you don't have a medical disease, then you don't have a clinical problem."

For each of the seventy-eight, I had recorded the essential facts on a 3x5 file card. For several weeks, I thumbed through the cards trying to find some method to group patients with similar characteristics. At first, it seemed I had accumulated a series of chaotic clinical experiences. However, I knew each patient extremely well; visions and memories of my encounters came to mind as I examined each card. I tried defining groups by the number of symptoms; that led nowhere. I attempted to use duration of symptoms; that was not revealing. Using no preconceived logic or defined characteristic but instead a kind of overall gestalt, I starting dealing the cards into two piles, A and B. Soon I had divided the entire group of seventy-eight patients into piles of A-ness and B-ness. I began reflecting on what characteristics made a patient A rather than B. It became apparent that those in A generated warmer feelings than those in B. I felt more rewarded for my efforts. There was a heavy element of cooperativeness for the patients in A.

I went back through the records of each patient in the A and B groups and made additional notes. I had kept very complete records on all of them. I began to see that the patients in A were more aware of their surroundings, especially their associates and family. Eventually I made a finer cut and separated A into Groups I and II and B into Groups III and IV. I discovered that I had based my groupings on the patient's manner of presenting himself or herself in the initial visits. Here is how I eventually defined the four groups:

Group I.    The patient gives psychological or social information first, followed by the physical symptoms, in the first interview. The patient believes that life stress is causing the symptoms.

Group II.    The patient gives physical symptoms first, followed by psychological or social information, in the first interview. The patient *wonders* if life stress may be causing the symptoms but is not sure.

Group III. The patient gives only physical symptoms throughout the first interview. The patient gives psychological or social information in the second interview, but
only when directly requested. The patient admits to
some life stress but denies any possibility of its causing the symptoms.

Group IV. The patient gives only physical symptoms throughout the first two interviews. The patient passes over
psychological or social information, and also ig-
nores requests for it. The patient firmly denies any
life stress or even the possibility of its relationship to
any symptom.

The brief case reports that follow illustrate the characteristics of
the four patient groupings.

## Group I: Carolyn Anderson

Carolyn Anderson is a forty-five-year-old mother of two daughters.
The first thing she told me was that she had just moved to town following a contested divorce from her husband. The ex-husband had
gained custody of the children. Mrs. Anderson was now in a new
job, and in a new town, without her children.

She later said in the same interview that while all of these
events were occurring, she developed recurring nausea, diffuse abdominal pain, low back pain, and intense fatigue. She had gained
forty pounds in one year. She said, "There is no doubt in my mind
that all of this is pulling me down. I just wanted a medical check to
see if I had gone into some disease that needs treatment." She denied feeling depressed and lacked nearly all the other symptoms of
depression.

Comments: Following a discussion of her negative examination and of tests I had ordered, Mrs. Anderson said, "I'm glad to

know that I don't have some disease. I'll work it out all right. If I need you I'll call." A letter from her several months later described her general good health and a weight loss of ten pounds from her exercise and dieting efforts. None of the five patients in Group I carried a diagnosis of a disease. All five achieved symptom relief.

I suspect many people fit this category but never seek medical attention. Most people under stress know to get more rest, talk it over with a friend, go on a vacation, or take some other corrective action to avoid becoming sick.

## Group II: Lonzo Craig

Lonzo Craig is a thirty-eight-year-old truck driver whose initial complaints included dizziness, episodes of sweating, intermittent diarrhea, pounding in the chest (tachycardia), and feelings of weakness. He had been referred to me with a diagnosis of hypoglycemia. He had been advised to follow a high-protein diet and to eat often. The changed diet had not led to any improvement in his symptoms. Toward the end of the first interview he said, "You know, if that doctor hadn't told me I had low sugar, I would have sworn my wife and that new truck driver brought this on me." He went on to describe a wife who had found her independence and no longer cleaned his home as he thought it should be. His newly assigned truck-driving partner spent his time either cursing or trying to involve Mr. Craig with waitresses at every truck stop. Mr. Craig held strict religious views against profanity and "womanizing."

Mr. Craig did not have demonstrated hypoglycemia on repeated studies. He clearly saw some relationship between his profane new job partner, his changed wife, and his symptoms. However, he had been diverted by the diagnosis of hypoglycemia. I suggested he keep daily notes about his symptoms and the circumstances of their occurrence. Within a month, he had had a long talk with his wife and reconciled some of their differences. He asked for and got a transfer back to his old driving partner. His symptoms disappeared completely and he was eating candy bars again and enjoying them.

Comment: Patients in Group II had not made a clear association between their symptoms and their lives. As with Mr. Craig, the patients in Group II freely discussed their social or psychological situations within the first two visits. Eleven of the twenty patients in Group II carried diagnoses of nonexistent diseases. With coaching, all the diagnoses were removed. With some personal effort and further observations by the patients, all twenty achieved symptom relief.

## Group III: Christine Swanson

Christine Swanson, a twenty-seven-year-old secretary, was single. She initially complained of having had diarrhea for three years and of a slow weight loss of fifteen pounds. She had been hospitalized twice. On the first hospitalization, she was told she had gallbladder disease, and her gallbladder was removed. The diarrhea continued. On a second hospitalization, she had an extensive workup for gastrointestinal malabsorption, including a small bowel biopsy. She then changed physicians and was told she had either ulcerative colitis or Crohn's disease. She had read extensively about ulcerative colitis and asked me about total and partial removal of her colon. On the second interview, she admitted having some problems with her boss, whom she said she hated. She said, "But none of that has anything to do with my colitis."

A review of her outside radiologic studies and test results together with a repeat barium enema, an endoscopic examination of her colon, and tests for occult blood in her stools were all negative.

I suggested Christine keep a diary and record each stool, its place and time of occurrence, its relation to meals, and the content of each meal. She spent two weeks focusing on food and even tried eliminating milk and a variety of other foods. She also reported that the diarrhea was less on the weekend when she saw her lover and worse during the week. A few weeks later, she discussed a correlation between her diarrhea and the intensity of her perceived conflict with her boss. This conflict centered on (1) her need for a job so she could continue her night college work and (2) her knowledge of her boss's alleged embezzling. If she reported him, she would lose her job and income, and she also feared his threats to involve her in his crime. If she did not report him, she would continue to feel guilty and unworthy.

After several months, Christine quit her job and reported her boss to the president of the company. Within a month, the diarrhea ceased and she remained free of it over the year I continued to hear from her.

Comment: This patient, as was characteristic of the twenty-four patients in Group III, at first saw no relationship between her life situation and her symptoms. Ten of the twenty-four patients in Group III carried diagnoses of nonexistent diseases. The diagnoses diverted attention from the real underlying causes. It was only with repeated careful directed observations, for example, that Christine uncovered what she thought was her underlying problem. She then took action, which resolved her dilemma and her diarrhea.

Of the ten patients with medical diagnoses in Group III, I was able to persuade eight that they did not have the diagnosed disease. Two persisted in hanging on to the diagnosis of the nonexistent disease and were lost to my follow-up. About half the Group III patients achieved symptom relief.

## Group IV: Sarah Madison

Sarah Madison was a forty-four-year-old married mother of three adult children. Her major complaint was back pain of five years' duration. In addition, she complained of fatigue, inability to do housework, abdominal pains, chest pains, severe constipation, frontal headaches, and buzzing in her ears. In her past, she had a hysterectomy, removal of her gallbladder, two uterine dilatation and curettages, and two breast biopsies. She was taking five medicines daily. She told me she had a herniated disc that had "eat up the nerves in my back." In addition to an extensive medical workup, she had two normal spinal myelograms. She had been seen by many specialists, but no medical diagnosis had been made. I found no medical disease with my workup.

At no time in the first two interviews did Mrs. Madison mention any problems with her family or children. She described them as "wonderful and loving." Her husband later told me that his wife's trouble got worse when their daughter had an illegitimate child. Another daughter divorced and moved back into the home with her parents. The son and his wife were contemplating moving back into his parents' home so they "could be with their sick mother."

I offered to see Mrs. Madison for a limited six visits if she would keep a diary of her symptoms and try to make correlations with any aggravating factors. She called to break the first two appointments. Her husband called several weeks later to tell me his wife was worse than ever and had been admitted to another hospital. Her new doctor had just told them he was probably going to fuse her spine. I never heard from the patient again.

Comment: Mrs. Madison's refusal to attempt to observe her life and her symptoms is characteristic of the twenty-nine patients in this group. Not only do Group IV patients deny any life stress, they deny any possibility of a relationship between their life and their health. Of the twenty-nine patients in Group IV, twenty-one carried a diagnosis of a nonexistent disease. I was able to convince only four that they did not have the diagnosed disease (Florence in Chapter 10 was one of them). Seventeen of the twenty-one continued to take medicines and to believe they had the diagnosed disease (Sweet Thing in Chapter 8 was one of these). Only three patients, including Florence, achieved symptom relief.

## Self-Awareness, Connection to Life, and Willingness to Explore

The method of grouping I used is not a diagnostic tool nor does it substitute for a thorough medical workup. Keep in mind that I created the groupings only after medical diagnoses had been excluded by extensive testing. The groupings describe some characteristics of a special subset of patients who presented with symptoms but who did not have a demonstrable disease to explain them. The method also does not predict the presence or absence of psychological or social stress. It is a scale of the patient's awareness of self and surroundings, connectedness to life, and willingness to participate in teasing out causative associations (see Table 11-1).

Although a patient readily admits to stress (Group I) and believes the stress explains the symptoms, there still needs to be a medical evaluation to exclude likely diseases. Even though in these groupings I used the timing with which patients introduced social and psychological information (that is, in their first or second vis-

Table 11-1. Grouping of Patients with Symptoms
Without Medical Disease

|  | Group I | Group II | Group III | Group IV |
|---|---|---|---|---|
| **Level of self-awareness** | Aware | Aware | Unaware | Unaware |
| **Level of connection of self to life** | Connected | Almost connected | Un-connected | Un-connected |
| **Level of willingness to explore life** | Willing | Willing | Willing | Unwilling |

its, or not at all), I do not mean to imply that all such patients have a psychological or social reason for their symptoms. Finding the real causative or triggering factors for any symptom takes collaboration between the physician and the patient. For patients who fall into Groups I, II, or even III, the collaborative effort to trace causation will likely be productive. For patients with the characteristics of Group IV, the effort will be largely futile. Maybe future studies and research of this group of patients will lead to more productive approaches than I was able to find.

Although I did not test the idea systematically, I found this method for grouping by awareness and connectedness to life events also useful for patients with a defined medical disease. Even though I did not subject the excluded seventy-two patients to detailed analysis, it was my experience that patients who fell into Groups I, II, or III were more amenable to examining their daily lives, even when there was a medical disease present. They were amenable to changing habits, making adjustments in their lives, and taking medications that the disease process required for maximum improvement.

For patients with the characteristics of Group IV, disease is a way of life whether it is objectively demonstrable or not. I believe, but cannot prove, that patients with the characteristics of Group IV will do more poorly with medical diseases than those in Groups I, II, or III. Some patients in Group IV "use" their diseases to manipulate their families and friends.

## "Diagnoses" Not Found

Of the seventy-eight patients with symptoms but no diagnosable disease, there were sixty-one women and seventeen men. Forty-one of the patients carried diagnoses of nonexistent diseases. Forty-six had had surgical procedures. Seventeen of the sixty-one women had had a hysterectomy. There were 165 previous surgical operations among the seventy-eight patients, an average of 2.1 operations per patient.

One of the most telling aspects of this study is the number and nature of the false diagnoses carried by these patients. Table 11-2 lists the forty-two diagnoses that were not substantiated by further study. Aside from diverting the attention of patients from the real source of their problems, some of these labels are serious and harmful enough to be worthy of comment. Some are frightening.

Florence, as we have seen, was told she had a detaching retina. Another patient was told the lipoma on her forearm was potentially malignant. An older woman was told she had a cerebral aneurysm. Two were told they had strokes. Still another was told that she had a malignant lymphoma.

Two patients were taking propylthiouracil for unsubstantiated hyperthyroidism. Sweet Thing was taking insulin for her misdiagnosed diabetes and having frequent hypoglycemic episodes.

One patient was referred for cobalt therapy to the pituitary gland for a false diagnosis of acromegaly. The diagnosis was based on borderline physical findings of a large face, jaw, and hands, and a growth-hormone level at the upper limits of normal that allegedly was not suppressed with glucose administration. When I questioned the patient, she said she had not received any glucose on the day of the serial measurements. An infusion of glucose produced complete suppression of her growth-hormone levels.

One patient had had serial teeth extractions until all the teeth had been removed from the entire left side of her mouth. There were two patients on glucocorticoids for false diagnoses of thyroiditis. One patient was on chronic coumadin therapy for "phlebitis," which turned out to be self-produced bruises along the course of the veins in her legs.

Most of the false diagnoses in the patients I saw concerned endocrine diseases, because this was my specialty practice. I suspect

Table 11-2. "Diagnoses" Not Found among 78 Patients
with Symptoms without Medical Diseases

Group I    None

Group II    Diabetes mellitus (not on insulin)
Duodenal ulcer
Hyperthyroidism (on propylthiouracil)
Hypoglycemia (3)
Lipomata (fatty-tissue tumor), possibly malignant
Multiple allergies
Ovarian failure
Sinusitis
Ulcerative colitis or Crohn's Disease

Group III    Acromegaly (excess growth hormone)
Congenital heart disease
Diabetes mellitus (on 20 units insulin daily)
Hiatus hernia
Hypertension
Hypoglycemia
Hypothyroidism
Rheumatoid arthritis
Ulcerative colitis
Uterine tumor

Group IV    Abscess of teeth
Bladder obstruction (3)
Cerebral aneurysm
Coronary artery disease
"Detaching" retina
Duodenal ulcer
Heart failure
Hiatus hernia (2)
Hyperthyroidism (on propylthiouracil)
Lymphoma
Migraine headaches
Multiple allergies
Stroke (2)
Thrombophlebitis
Thyroiditis (2)
Ulcerative colitis

but cannot prove that the diagnosis of similar patients from different specialists' practices would reflect the diseases seen in those specialties. Clearly, the false diagnoses had the potential to produce serious and harmful consequences, both psychologically and physically.

## Prevalence of False Diagnoses: An Unanswered Question

One of the questions I posed in the introduction to this book was, "How common is the error of assigning a false diagnosis to a patient?" In attempting to answer this question, I have searched the literature every few years since 1965. I have found only one study that defined the extent of false diagnoses of a disease in a population, and that tracked the number of false diagnoses of heart disease in 20,000 school children in Seattle. Bergman and Stamm (1967) found 110 children with a diagnosis of heart disease who were then subjected to detailed cardiac evaluation. Only 18 percent actually had heart disease; 72 percent had no heart disease. If false diagnoses of other chronic diseases are even close to this magnitude, there is obviously a serious problem in the health-care system.

Since 1967, I have been unable to find another population-based study that attempted to define the prevalence of any false diagnosis. The literature is full of studies of the errors of missing diagnoses of all sorts. Yet the unaddressed and unanswered question remains: "What is the prevalence of false diagnoses of the major chronic diseases?" It is an idea that can and should be addressed by a properly designed epidemiological study of patients who carry diagnoses of the major medical diseases. I remain puzzled by the complete lack of attention to this problem.

I coauthored an article in 1995 titled "The Cryptic Error of Nondisease: The Hidden Power of Prevalence of Disease" (Meador and Lanius 1995) that attempted to present a testable theory to explain this lack of interest and attention. The paper to my knowledge has itself received no attention.

• • •

After 1976, I began to expand my practice to problem patients of all sorts. The principles and techniques I used in this series of seventy-eight patients proved useful in a variety of patient problems. I also began to add other methods and techniques to my interviewing, listening, and communication strategies, as the case reports in the chapters to follow demonstrate.

# 12
# Looking Back on Fairhope

In 1981, my medical odyssey took me to Fairhope, Alabama. Each Friday, four or five clinical faculty members flew in the university airplane out into the small towns of south Alabama to give lectures, demonstrations, and consultations to practicing physicians. Late in the afternoon, after the faculty members had been picked up, each from a different town, we flew south down the branching and converging waters of the rivers north of Mobile. The waters glistened and broadened, eventually forming the backwaters and then the expanse of Mobile Bay that stretched more than thirty miles to the Gulf of Mexico. To our right was the port of Mobile. Far off in the distance to the east, we saw the jut of land called Fairhope.

The pilot, something of a daredevil, then turned the plane into a sharply descending dive, swooping to within fifty feet of the waters of the bay. We flew at that level toward the eastern shore. Shortly, we neared the rows of sticklike piers in front of hundreds of clapboard summer homes. We aimed at the pier where we knew our wives were gathered to wave at us as we returned from our day in the field. Just as we roared over the pier, the plane abruptly rose and tipped its wings to the gathering below. The wives waved back, signaling a weekend of parties, sun, boat rides, and seafood.

In 1894, a group of farmers and citizens from Iowa formed a commune and colony in what is now Fairhope. Supporters of a national single-tax movement, their dream was to have a single tax and live in a community with joint ownership of the land. They wrote back to family in Iowa, "There is a fair hope that our experiment will work"—hence the name of the town. In the long run, the single-tax movement failed, but the community thrived. I thought Fairhope was a name of promise for a sabbatical adventure. I wanted to find out what really goes on between patients and physicians.

The winds and breezes that blow across ten miles of water make the eastern shore of Mobile Bay much cooler than the surrounding land and therefore perfect for a summer home. In the 1890s, many families from Mobile built summer homes along the bay shore from Fairhope to Point Clear. The fathers went back and forth to their work in Mobile by large paddleboats. The small town of Fairhope over the years has become a haven for artists, writers, and eccentrics of all sorts. It is a community of intellectuals and thus was an ideal setting for the work of H. C. "Moon" Mullins, family physician and longtime personal friend.

Moon, as everyone called him, was a visionary but also a man of action. He had accepted the chair of the newly formed Department of Family Medicine at the University of South Alabama School of Medicine in Mobile. Family medicine in academic circles was still a new specialty, and Moon set out to build an outstanding department. Recalling my own days as a dean when I struggled with what to do about incorporating family medicine, I also wanted to find out what the specialty was all about.

Moon had practiced family medicine for more than twenty years and knew intuitively that medicine at its heart had to encompass human communication. As soon as he became chair of the department, he recruited an outstanding team of behavioral scientists. When I heard of his efforts, I immediately made plans to spend my sabbatical with Moon and his team.

In addition to gathering the team of behavioral scientists, Moon had built a near state-of-the-art audiovisual recording facility in the clinic building in Fairhope. This teaching clinic was remote from the main campus in Mobile, but it provided a laboratory for more ordinary types of clinical problems. All the patients were patients of Moon and his three partners. The clinic was their practice site. The recording facilities were attached to the clinic. There were one-way mirrors, conference rooms, extensive audiovisual recording equipment, and everything one might need to observe and record interactions between doctors and patients.

To supplement the stationary recording equipment in the clinic, we soon built portable enclosures, crude folding panels that we could fit into the corners of any exam room, two to a room. These we took out into the physicians' offices in small towns across south Alabama.

Moon had recruited Stonewall Stickney, a psychiatrist and former commissioner of the state mental health system for Alabama. "Stone," as we called him, was one of a kind. He was analytically trained and extraordinarily well-read both in psychiatry and in world literature. He was constantly reciting or making up limericks. Above all, he had an uncanny ability to get to the core of a person's psychological makeup.

The other two members of the team, in addition to me, were Joseph and Susan Conley. Susan F. Conley had completed work on her doctoral degree in animal behavior, specializing in observing foxes. Almost all of what I say here about the analysis of our recordings comes from Susan's observations. Joseph C. Conley, her husband, did his graduate work in clinical psychiatric social work. He, like Stone, was extremely well-read, particularly in Freud. He too was intuitive and could get to the heart of a clinical problem quickly.

We spent months attempting to videotape full encounters between patients and physicians in the clinic. This was in the early days of videotape recordings, and we had constant equipment failures of all kinds. Often either the patient or the physician would move off camera. The equipment was not yet remote, so we had two people in the exam room behind wooden blinds to run the cameras. In addition to the two cameras in the room, we had a third wide-angle camera in a cut-through in the wall to capture both the physician and the patient, feet to head, in the same recorded view.

The problems in the offices of private physicians were even more formidable. We never got a recording of a complete encounter in the field. Eventually, we finally got one full recording of one patient and one physician at the main clinic. The tape lasted only 157 seconds. This one recording became the focus of our efforts for the next several months. Susan spent more than sixty hours moving the video frames back and forth, noting every movement and verbalization of both the physician and the patient, along with the time interval of the movement. She then transcribed the sequence so we could read serially what the patient did and said and what the physician did and said. The level of detail was remarkable. Susan was in effect creating a dictionary of minute doctor and patient behaviors. She then noted what she called utterances, classifying each utterance and noting its time intervals. Our intent was to categorize with no preconceptions what we saw and heard. Susan and Joe refused to theorize about what we observed. They wanted to build our studies through phases of direct observations. "Watching and wondering" was the byword of ethologists (animal behaviorists) of that day. Susan categorized every slight movement, tone of voice, inflection, and utterance. Her dictionary of behaviors ran well over fifty pages, all from the 157-second tape.

Even though Susan and Joe refused to speculate, Stone and I spent hours theorizing about what we observed on the tapes and about the clustered behaviors that Susan had teased out. Most of our conjectures came from our observations through the one-way mirrors. Stone might say, as we watched a doctor and patient, "What do you make of that?' Or I would say, "Did you catch that head nod just before he asked about chest pain?" "Did you notice he did not see the patient frowning since his head was buried in the medical record?" "Did you notice how he phrased that question anticipating a positive answer?"

During my sabbatical, I read extensively the writings of John Grinder and Richard Bandler. They introduced me to the ideas of unspecified language and methods for establishing rapport, particularly the notion of people having verbal, visual, or kinesthetic representational systems. I also learned to pay attention to the verbs patients used and to their facial expressions (Bandler and Grinder 1976a, 1976b, 1979). Grinder and Bandler modeled many of their ideas from careful observations of Milton Erickson, a psychiatrist and superb therapeutic hypnotist (Bandler and Grinder 1982; Haley 1986, 1987; Erickson and Rossi 1979). The appeal of their ideas is that they are stated in terms that can be refuted by direct observation—thus they are subject to scientific study. No one has yet done such a study, and the writings of both authors remain outside the mainstream medical literature. In many of the cases that follow in this book, I use techniques that came from the ideas of these authors.

Stonewall Stickney and I made some tentative observations and speculations from our experiences. I say "tentative" because we did not conduct full-fledged scientific experiments. We did not do field experiments with the physicians, having them, for example, redirect their cued statements to test the notion of cuing.

In one observation, we noticed a lot of movement (hands, arms, head, feet, breathing, eyeblinks) going on by and between patient and doctor. Sometimes these movements of the physician were copied by the patient and a synchrony developed. We speculated that when the patient copies a movement of the physician, the patient is in a receptive state for instructions. We called this a state of "attentive rapport."

In another observation, we saw that the physician preceded a lot of questions to the patient with a head nod (yes) or headshake (no). Often the physician phrased the question with an affirmative or negative direction. For example, a negative direction would be stated as, "You haven't had any nausea, have you?" The direction of the answers by the patients showed striking congruence with the direction of the question, that is, a "yes" direction of a question generated a "yes" answer; a "no" direction of a question generated a "no" answer. We speculated that the doctor was cuing the patient to answer questions along some preconceived lines of thought.

• • •

Cuing as a phenomenon has been well established in planned group experiments. Jerome Frank (Frank and Frank 1991) discusses it in some detail. There are many instances where cuing could be occurring between physician and patient, but none of these have been studied by direct observation. For instance, with cuing, informed consent could be directed and obtained without the patient's clear awareness. The physician could instill the correct way to take medication. The entire repertoire of Balint's apostolic functions, which I mention in the introduction, can be conveyed by cuing, and cuing is likely to establish the placebo effect. Unwittingly, negative outcomes and reactions can also be conveyed by cuing. According to Frank, cuing appears to occur beyond the awareness of the person being cued. Stickney came to believe that it is the principal method by which some if not many physicians convey information to patients.

I have come to believe that physicians call patients "difficult" when they refuse to be brought into a state of receptive rapport and thereby resist cuing. That is, they recoil, resist full rapport, object, or do whatever it takes to remain unreceptive to the physician. In simple terms, they will not listen or pay attention to the physician. The physician senses this resistance and rejects the patient. This idea also could be tested by direct observation.

Even though I have no proof of these theories, they fit and explain many of the experiences I have recorded in the chapters of this book. I have hesitated to include these conjectures because they are radical and heterodox. But I would not be true to myself or to Stonewall Stickney if I omitted them. I can only hope they will be put under scrutiny and substantiated or refuted by others.

Some widespread problems can come from the medical community's failure to accept the phenomenon of cuing. A good example of such problems lies in the use of informed consent for elective procedures. Informed consent obtained by the physician who will do the elective procedure is probably not truly informed consent. It is at best informed persuasion. I am so certain of this concern that I suggest that someone not doing or involved in the procedure should obtain the consent of the patient. The extreme variation in the rate of procedures across small geographic areas also suggests that some factor other than clinical need is operating (see Wennberg and Gittelsohn 1982). At the very least, to test these ideas, the profession should carefully study video-recorded examples of physicians obtaining informed consent.

•  •  •

Our Fairhope team was unable to obtain grant funds to continue our basic observations of doctors and patients. Several foundations said we provided no basis for our suggested studies. I have often wondered if behavioral studies of the sort we suggested were simply outside the prevailing biomolecular model and therefore not fundable. I hope the funding agencies have now moved beyond that point.

# 13
# The Diarrhea of Agnes

Agnes was referred to me by a physician from the next county. I had returned to Vanderbilt and Saint Thomas from my sabbatical in Fairhope, even more determined to explore and define the problems of patients with SUO. Agnes had suffered from chronic diarrhea for nearly a year. An extensive GI workup by her referring physician, including a small-bowel biopsy, was entirely normal. All symptomatic medicines had failed to produce any consistent relief. Every test I might consider had already been done, with negative findings. The results of the workup ruled out a long list of diseases, but it did not establish a diagnosis. Agnes had noted no pattern to the diarrhea and thought it came "all the time."

I had discovered through the years that almost no symptom comes "all the time." I had learned to gently challenge that statement by saying, "By 'all the time,' I am wondering if you mean every minute of every day and every night?" Note how I embedded the challenge in a question. Embedding challenges in questions reduces the chance of a defensive answer. People hear embedded challenges as less confrontational than direct challenges.

Agnes's answer was quick. "Well, no. Not all the time. It comes and goes." There had to be a pattern of some sort. All symptoms wobble, vary, and come and go. The trick is to get the patient to find and define that wobble, that variance. Insistence by a patient that any chronic symptom is continuous or "all the time" is a red flag. By challenging Agnes, I was setting in motion a search for the pattern of the diarrhea. She did not know her pattern of diarrhea on the early visits and would have to discover it.

I had found my approach of refusing to label patients prematurely more and more useful and productive. I said to Agnes, as Sapira taught me, "I don't know what you have . . . *yet.*" Again, I emphasized the "yet." I also continued to list for patients many of the diseases I knew were absent. I was careful to name those diseases that had killed some member of the family if I was sure the patient did not have that disease. My reasoning was that whatever buried anxiety patients might have had over the family "killer" might be reduced by specifically telling them the disease was not present. In some cases, I suspected that the anxiety and worry over inheriting a family disease were sufficient in themselves to produce the symptoms. My statement at least got the subject out in the open in a subtle manner. For Agnes, there were no family killers of note. Both parents were still alive and all grandparents lived into old age.

With Agnes, as with other patients, I wanted to avoid using what I call "dead-end diagnoses." Such labels inhibit all etiological thinking by the physician and the patient. In a case like Agnes's, examples of dead-end diagnoses are spastic colon, irritable bowel, and sometimes diverticulosis. Without exhaustive examinations for causes, these labels are prematurely definitive. Something, usually something ingested, is causing the bowel to be irritable or the colon to be spastic. Why not try to identify it? That was the direction of my thinking with Agnes.

I came to my two favorite questions. I asked Agnes: "What are you doing that you should stop doing? Or what should you be doing that you are not doing?"

With more and more experience with patients, I was becoming extremely careful in my choice of words. Notice that both questions leave out all specific detail. There was no mention of time or place or context, yet both questions clearly directed the patient to do an exhaustive mental search. The command was embedded in the unspecified language. I was directing the patient to search for an answer, but I was not specifying in any way what area of life was to be scanned. In the first question, I left open all possibilities for what actions the patient could stop doing. In the second question, I left open all possibilities for what actions should be added to the patient's life. These directed but unspecified injunctions create maximum internal mental searches for answers. They leave all content to the patient. There is a certain elegance in using a process approach such as this and staying out of content. As long as the process leads to corrective action, I do not need to know the content. The patient most certainly does. This approach also permits the patient to find or admit to hidden perverse or abhorrent behaviors without discussing them. The method certainly honors the personal integrity of the patient.

This notion of "contentless" inquiry bears some emphasis. By using unspecified language, the physician stays out of content. The patient therefore *must* try to make sense out of the questions. He or she *must* go within to seek answers. This powerful technique clearly pushes the patient to find solutions, as specified and direct questions do not. Real information comes when the physician stays away from defining, directing, or in any way limiting the subject-matter focus of the patient's mental exploration as he or she (not the physician) searches for answers.

I was also becoming more aware of the timing of my words and the inflections of my voice. In both these questions, I emphasize certain short phrases with my tone: "What are you doing that you should *stop doing*?" Said in this manner, the question is an injunction—a very subtle doctor's order. I supposed the brain would hear this as "stop doing" whatever it had sorted out to be stopped. For the second question, I emphasize with my tone of voice and volume "*should be doing*," making this an injunction for the patient to discover what action might be missing. I had learned to wait after each injunction. I took my cue from the facial expressions of the patient. Either question could produce deep thought with slackened facial muscles and sometimes a drooping of the mouth. I waited as long as necessary until the patient shifted to a more alert facial expression. Sometimes this took a minute or more.

My intention was to leave the door open to all possibilities by being directive but not specific. I wanted the patient to supply the specificity from his or her own thoughts and observations, not from mine. If I asked specific questions, the patient could only affirm or deny them. If I ask, "Do you have a pain in your upper stomach area?" the patient can answer either yes or no. I am literally guessing when I ask narrow questions, and guessing can go on ad infinitum. However, if I ask the question more broadly—"Do you ever have any pains?"—then I have opened up the whole of the human body for the patient to scan mentally. Thus, if I ask general nonspecified questions, the patient must supply the detail. To do so, a patient must use his or her mind. Unspecified questions, well put, are like the scanning dials on radios. Specified questions are like dialing to a single radio station.

With Agnes, in addition to the two unspecified questions, I asked her to note in a diary the time and place of each bowel movement and the associations that came to mind. I had her add a number of other columns for observations she might wish to make. I asked Agnes to make an entry every four to six hours. (For patients with frequently occurring symptoms, I suggested making entries every hour or so.) Agnes's diary revealed a late-morning and late-evening pattern to her diarrhea.

I also suggested that Agnes do little experiments. I suggested she try to do something that would make the symptom worse and try to do something that would alleviate the symptom. (Again note my unspecified language: "do something.") Either bit of information would be useful. Paradoxically, one of the most powerful bits of information comes when a patient finds something that will aggravate a symptom. At the least, it gives the patient a sense of control, often when none was present before. At its full power, the discovery can lead to a method to eliminate the symptom.

Agnes did her "little experiment," as she called it. She omitted breakfast and still had the late morning diarrhea. She then omitted supper and still had the nighttime diarrhea that woke her around 2:30 in the morning. The plot clearly thickened. I could not figure it out at all.

On the next visit, Agnes had a big clue and nearly the answer. She omitted brushing her teeth and there was no diarrhea. Her GI tract had to be reacting to something in her toothpaste. I suggested she switch brands (she was using Crest toothpaste). When she did, the diarrhea vanished. Several weeks later, I asked that she go back to Crest and the diarrhea reappeared. "Crest toothpaste diarrhea," of all things. I had never heard of it.

After I referred her back to her physician, I asked that she write me a card from time to time. I heard from her on several occasions. Agnes remained free of diarrhea. I last heard from her two years later.

I have no idea what is in Crest toothpaste that caused Agnes to have diarrhea. I have not seen another case of it, although I have asked many patients with diarrhea about their use of toothpaste since then. None of them found any correlation with the brand of toothpaste.

For patients with chronic symptoms, it is important to remain open to any causative agent as a possibility. The use of the unspecified questions directed Agnes to search, and the symptom diary provided her a method to record her observations. I did have Agnes challenge herself with Crest toothpaste, and the recurrence of diarrhea nailed down the diagnosis.

I am sure there are clinical trial purists out there who will say I should have double-blinded the study by putting the toothpaste brands in containers marked only A or B. But I was after only symptom relief. Clinical medicine can sometimes stop short of scientific certainty.

•  •  •

Some patients have their own idiosyncratic disease. Premature use of loose diagnostic terms such as "spastic colon" or "irritable bowel" precludes finding such idiosyncratic causes. All symptoms are stimulated or provoked by something. The trick is to find the trigger. It is not always possible, but the pursuit is worth the time and effort.

# 14
# Dr. Jim's Breasts

There is an old dictum that the patient will tell you what is wrong with him if you listen carefully. That rule was reinforced by my experience with Dr. Jim.

I had known Dr. Jim for many years. He practiced in a small town not too far from Nashville, where I now saw patients alongside my teaching duties. He had sent me a number of patients through the years. Now seventy-six years old, he was complaining of breast enlargement. The enlargement had started in the right breast. Because the enlargement was unilateral, it was thought he might have cancer of the breast. The right breast had been removed surgically before Dr. Jim asked me to see him. Cancer of the male breast is not a common lesion, but it can be quite malignant when it does occur.

Examination of the tissue did not show cancer but showed typical changes of gynecomastia (enlargement of the male breast). These changes are indicative of estrogen stimulation. (The normally dormant male breast can be converted to a fully functioning "female breast" if the proper mix of female hormones is present in the bloodstream.) The finding of unilateral gynecomastia was puzzling, and it was after that finding that Dr. Jim asked to see me. His left breast had now begun to enlarge.

I was not too confounded by the initial unilaterality because I had seen that before. There is sometimes a lag in the response of the breasts, and one will enlarge before the other even though the female hormone is available to both breasts. What did concern me was the appearance of gynecomastia at Dr. Jim's age. It usually meant the presence of a malignant tumor of the testicle or the adrenal.

The normal male at puberty secretes both female hormone and male hormone. Enlargement of the breasts in teenage boys is nearly universal if you palpate carefully. This early influence of the female hormone is soon replaced with the dominance of the male hormone, which is secreted in increasing amounts. The effect of the female hormone is inhibited, and the breast enlargement is suppressed. At any time in later life, this balance can be upset. If enough female hormone is present, breast enlargement will occur in a male of any age.

In the adult male, there are only two endogenous sources of female hormones—the testicles and the adrenal glands. Both normally secrete very small amounts of estrogens. Both, however, can develop tumors that are capable of secreting large amounts of estrogens. That was my first concern, because these tumors are highly malignant, that is, they grow and spread rapidly. There is a very narrow window of time when surgical removal is still curative. (This was before effective chemotherapy was available for any of these tumors.)

There is one other rare cause of estrogen secretion in the adult male: malignant tumors of various organs that curiously begin to make pituitarylike hormones that stimulate the adrenal or testicle to secrete estrogens. Lung cancer, for instance, can produce this bizarre biochemical aberration.

Turning to the case of Dr. Jim, with these ominous and very serious possibilities of cancers in mind, I ordered all the tests that would identify the presence of estrogens or the hormones that can stimulate estrogen production. All the tests showed the very low and normal levels of estrogens typical for a man his age. What a surprise! Knowing that false negative results can occur, I repeated the tests. Again, the results came back within normal limits for a male.

My initial physical examination had been normal except for the easily felt gynecomastia of the remaining breast. I repeated the physical examination, this time giving extra time and attention to palpating Dr. Jim's testicles for masses and pushing here and there in his abdomen trying to feel his deep-seated adrenals. My examination was normal again. (This case occurred before abdominal CAT scans were available.)

Not satisfied with these normal results and still quite concerned that there was a malignant tumor hidden away somewhere, I began to do x-rays and other procedures to find a tumor. I reasoned that there are numerous compounds that can have an estrogen effect. The tests available measured only a small number of these compounds. Dr. Jim could be secreting a "hybrid" estrogen, if you will, and thus appear to have normal levels because the tests I ordered were not "seeing" the novel hormone. It was a bit of fancy thinking, but I did not want to miss a malignancy that might still be surgically removable.

All the imaging tests and procedures showed no tumors. I was up a blind alley and baffled. I had a colleague see Dr. Jim with me in consultation. He had no new thoughts but suggested repeating the tests once more, which we did—only to find the same normal results.

I then recalled a patient I had seen years before. He was a young boy about six years old who had developed gynecomastia at age five. Gynecomastia at that age is as ominous as at Dr. Jim's age. The list of possibilities is as full of cancers if not more so. After an exhaustive but negative search for tumors in the boy, I began to look around for other causes. I had his mother bring in all the medicines in the house, thinking that the boy might be getting into her birth-control pills or some estrogen-type compound. The only medicine at all was a vitamin the boy took on a routine basis. I had hit a dead-end.

A few months later, there was a report in a medical journal that a certain brand of vitamins had been contaminated with estrogens.

Apparently, in the process of stamping, the same press used to make estrogen pills was used to press out the vitamin pills. Enough estrogen was carried over on the press to contaminate the vitamins. I immediately thought of the little boy who had me so puzzled, and I called his mother. Sure enough, the vitamins were the same brand. Stopping the vitamins led to a regression of the little boy's breasts back to normal within a few months. I was amazed at how such a minute dose of estrogen could produce such a profound physical effect.

When I thought of the little boy, I called Dr. Jim. I had taken a careful drug history when I first saw him and got no clue that he was taking anything that might have estrogen in it. I had even gotten the nerve to ask him if he smoked marijuana, a frequent cause of gynecomastia in the drug subculture. After he laughed at my question, he asked me if I thought he was one of "those long-haired dope fiends." I asked if his wife took any estrogens, thinking somehow they might rub off on something he was using. I was fishing for any clue. He answered that she was not taking any.

I told him the story of the little boy and the contaminated vitamins. I asked him to see if he could come up with anything he was doing or taking that could stimulate the breasts to enlarge. I suggested that Dr. Jim keep a diary. He laughed and rejected the notion as silly.

I didn't see Dr. Jim for more than a month. We had agreed to go along and see what happened. I was not at all satisfied with failing to make a diagnosis for such an obvious and ominous abnormality. One day, Dr. Jim showed up with his wife without an appointment. He was grinning and blurted out, "This was just too good to tell you over the phone. Gladys has made the diagnosis that you and I missed. Tell him, Gladys."

She went into great detail about their sex lives, how they had continued to "enjoy" each other frequently, sometimes several times a week. And then came the answer to the puzzle. For years, she had used a vaginal cream for an atrophic vaginitis (a condition in older women due to the absence of estrogen) and as a lubricant. Not knowing what was in the cream, she began to check around after I asked Dr. Jim to keep a diary. Sure enough, this cream commonly prescribed to postmenopausal women for atrophic vaginitis contained estrogen. Then she said, winking, "You don't suppose that has anything to do with Jim's breasts, do you?" And then she laughed out loud.

I just shook my head in disbelief. "We will certainly find out," I answered.

She had hit the diagnosis right on target. I knew the minute she told the story that she was right. Over several years, Dr. Jim must have absorbed enough estrogen through the skin to produce breast enlargement but not enough to measure in the tests. The couple stopped using the estrogen cream as a lubricant, and within a few months the remaining breast returned to normal.

Diseases can come from strange interactions between the infinite variety of stimuli from the world outside the body and the world of receptors inside the body. The trick in clinical medicine is to guide the patient to explore both worlds. I never in my wildest imagination would have thought of asking Dr. Jim if his wife was using vaginal estrogen cream.

• • •

It is awesome to consider the number of stimuli that exist in the world around us. Think just for a moment of the possible number of different substances we encounter in air and water. Add to that list plants, clothing, air conditioning, heating, food additives, dyes, soaps, lotions, and all the other compounds and chemicals— including vaginal estrogen creams. There is no way a physician or anyone else can think of all the possible toxic interactions that can occur. Then add to that perplexity the notion that each of us is biochemically and physiologically unique. One person's biochemical hell is another's heaven. What will make some of us sick will have no influence on others.

It is blatantly obvious that only the individual can begin to know the world around him or her. Certainly, others can direct the patient to look at this or examine that, but in the long run the person must figure out what is and is not affecting his or her health.

Again, I relearned what I had been taught earlier. Sooner or later, the patient will tell you what is wrong if you listen carefully— sometimes for a long time. And, I might add, it helps if patients are gently directed to look around themselves and wonder.

◆ ◆ ◆

After I made a brief report of Dr. Jim's breast in the *New England Journal of Medicine* (DiRaimondo, Roach, and Meador 1980), I got a call from Berton Roeuché, author of *Eleven Blue Men* and *Medical Detectives* (1947, 1988). He asked me about Dr. Jim's breast. I could not have been more surprised or pleased if Mark Twain had come to life and called me. Roeuché was a childhood hero of mine. I had read his stories over and over, saying to my father that I wanted to be the kind of doctor described in his stories. Roueché is best known for his medical detective stories, frequently published in the *New Yorker* magazine. On hearing of the case of Dr. Jim, Roueché visited me in Nashville and spent a day taking notes and gathering the details of the case. Sitting and talking with him that day was magical for me. He died before the case was published in the *New Yorker*; however, the case was published later in a book, *The Man Who Grew Two Breasts* (Roueché 1995).

I still puzzle over the irony and coincidence of finally meeting one of my early heroes and actually having him write up a case of mine and then name the book after my patient. It was one of the high points of my medical career to meet and get to know Berton Roueché, even though briefly. In some sense, the cases in this book are patterned after Roueché's methods of reporting. Mimicry, they say, is the highest form of flattery.

# 15
# The Woman
# Who Would Not Talk

I was asked to see Adelaine because of her diabetes mellitus. When I first saw her, she was a patient on the psychiatric unit in a state of severe depression. She had talked very little since admission and was about to receive electroshock therapy. I was asked to evaluate her medically prior to the electroconvulsive treatment. Adelaine was fifty-five years old, a widow, and the mother of one daughter, who lived nearby.

When I walked into her room, she was curled up in bed facing away from the door toward the window. I walked to the other side of the bed, pulled a chair to the bedside, and sat down facing her. She did not move but lay there with her eyes closed. I tried to get her to talk to me, but she did not move or respond in any manner. There was mention in the admission history of severe headaches of unknown duration but very little other detail. The daughter, who would later play an important role, had not yet come in to give the clinical history.

Adelaine had mild diabetes mellitus that was under fairly good control, with only mild blood-sugar elevations. Her physical examination was within normal limits, as were the remainder of her laboratory work and a chest x-ray. Skull x-rays and a spinal tap had been normal. A thorough neurological examination was within normal limits. I completed my physical examination, which was within normal limits except for her flaccid, withdrawn, and unresponsive state. She kept her eyes closed. During my examination, she did not say one word. I suspected she was more conscious and more present than she appeared. She winced with pain but did not withdraw when I gently pinched her arm.

I came back later that day. Puzzled by her withdrawn state and wanting to be sure I was not missing some other treatable internal disease, I sat and watched her for several minutes. I was trying to think through the situation. I could find no explanation for her clinical state from the laboratory or physical examination. The diabetes was not playing any significant role. I was confounded by the extreme state of her withdrawal and my continued belief that she was more conscious than she appeared. It somehow seemed too much or exaggerated. Depressed people are withdrawn but rarely to this degree.

To get a better look at her, I turned my head horizontally so that we were face to face. I bent slightly forward and put my head down on the mattress beside her pillow. I was trying to see if her face or her eyes were asymmetrical. I was still wondering if she had had a stroke. I stayed in this awkward position for a moment. Suddenly she opened her eyes and looked back at me. The sudden movement startled me. There I was with my head almost on the bed next to this curiously silent patient now staring back at me. I did not move but held the position.

I said, without moving my head, "Hello. How are you?"

She closed her eyes and slowly moved her head from side to side as if to say "no" or "not well." I was not sure what she meant. She said nothing, and the movement was ever so slight. I would have missed it if I had not been looking very closely. It was the kind of headshake that people who are very sick or nauseated make when they do not want to be bothered. She remained silent. Again I lay my head down on the bed beside her pillow. I wanted to see what would happen if I just stayed there. She looked directly at me and then moved her eyes down and away from me as if to avoid my eyes. Still holding my head sideways and on the bed, I took my finger and moved it in front of her eyes and she followed it in all the cardinal directions. All the complex neurological circuits that control eye movements were intact. There is a world of information in those six basic eye movements.

I had noted out of sheer happenstance with previous sick patients who lay on their sides in bed that I would unconsciously bend my head sideways. I did this to talk to them face to face rather than with their face at right angles to mine. Somehow and for unknown reasons, they seemed to respond to this position with more talk than if I kept my head vertical. I recalled these experiences with previous patients as I sat there with my head on the bed near Adelaine's pillow.

I continued to hold the position. I began to breathe in synchrony with Adelaine. I even tried to imagine what that degree of depression would feel like. I took a deep breath and noted that Adelaine did the same. I was in some curious synchrony with Adelaine. Then I slowly began to raise my head. To my amazement, Adelaine also began to raise her head. I very gradually continued to bring my head back to the vertical position, not saying a word but also not taking my gaze off her eyes, which were now wide open but looking downward. As I moved to a full sitting position in the chair, she gradually raised herself and swung her legs off the bed to a sitting position on the edge of the bed. She sank into a slumped position. Her head hung low between her shoulders. Her feet dangled off the edge of the bed. She braced herself with her hands on the bed. I was hesitant to say anything for fear of disrupting what was occurring. She sat there breathing heavily and sighing. I began to sigh, very slightly at first and then in synchrony with her. She nodded her head, eyes now closed, as if to say, "Yes, I know." She actually said nothing and did not look up. Obviously, I could only guess at what she meant by her head movements.

I could not see her face or her expressions so I bent very low until my head was under her face, in the position of looking under a table. From that awkward position, I looked up into her face. It was a ridiculous position, and I laughed without meaning to. She smiled faintly and very briefly.

I did not know what to do. I had no clear idea what was going on. I remember feeling confused, not having expected any of the things that had occurred. After a few moments, I asked her if she wanted me to leave. She shook her head no.

I sat by her bed in silence. For lack of anything else, I continued to breathe at the same depth and rate Adelaine did. When she sighed, I sighed. I kept at this for at least five minutes. Then I spent a few moments telling her all the negative findings of her laboratory work to that point. I told her I would discuss her situation with her psychiatrist. She showed no response to my monologue that I could detect. I then told her I had to leave but would return.

I called her psychiatrist. He did not know what to make of my encounter but encouraged me to visit her again to see if I could elicit any other responses. He agreed to delay the shock treatments until we had more information.

On my next visit with Adelaine, I was able to get her to copy the movements of my hands and body position. After I had breathed in synchrony with her for a few minutes, I noted that if I took a very deep breath, Adelaine also took a deep breath. That is when I moved my hand to a different position and she copied the movement. She also had begun to respond to my questions with a head-shake and to my laugh with a smile. I had no idea what she thought; I knew only that she was responding. My early efforts to get her to talk had been futile. On my next visit, I was more successful.

Here I want to warn you: I am recalling from memory what I think I said and did. Without a video and audio recording, I cannot be sure. My hope is that this account will provoke others to examine these techniques with other patients.

On my next visit, Adelaine was sitting on the bed. The nurse said she had mumbled some words, asked for water, and seemed to be responding to simple commands and requests from the nurses. I sat down and said nothing. Adelaine looked up at me.

I asked, "Can you tell me the story of your headaches?"

She shook her head no.

I said, "Maybe you can draw it out for me. I don't get a clear picture of your history."

Here I was trying first an auditory question with "tell." That failing, I went to visual words: "draw" and "clear picture." That too failed. Adelaine furrowed her brow to both attempts and slowly shook her head. I spent several more minutes trying visual and auditory commands and all failed to evoke anything except a headshake or a furrowed brow.

I made innumerable efforts, using visual and auditory commands and phrases, to try to get her to talk. I was consciously testing the notion that there are auditory and visual people. On failing with visual and auditory words and being as certain as possible that both would continue to fail to produce responses, I turned to kinesthetic or feeling-type phrases and verbs. I thought for a few moments how I might evoke kinesthetic processing on her part. Here is an approximation of what I said. This portion of my notes was written the day of the encounter while it was fresh in my memory.

"Try to *move* back into time. Let your mind and body *move* back along your memory. *Push* yourself to that place and *feel* what you were doing. *Feel* your feet *touching* what they were *touching. Stand* or *sit* where you were. *Feel* the air around you and the *temperature. Feel* your clothing."

I said as many feeling and movement and kinesthetic words as I could think of. I also, if you noticed, stayed unspecified in my choice of other words. I used generic terms, hoping she would supply the specific information. I was trying to get her to give me the history of the onset of her headaches using techniques described by Richard Bandler and John Grinder (1976a, 1976b, 1979, 1982).

A remarkable thing started to happen as I watched her face

and upper body. Her breathing became very slow and deep. All the muscles of her face relaxed. She looked like an entirely different person. The furrows on her brow disappeared. The wrinkles around her mouth smoothed out. Her facial color turned from a faint gray-green to a slight pink. The pulse rate in her neck slowed. She looked calm and relaxed, even pleased.

I felt a rush of excitement. Here this strange and almost un-believable model of communication appeared to be producing a response where all efforts before had failed.

There is a method described by Bandler and Grinder called "overlapping." Using this, one moves from one sensory modality to another as a way of helping a person fully develop the desired internal state, which for Adelaine was a recalled memory of the onset of her headaches. By overlapping, I mean that one moves from kinesthetic words to visual words to auditory words. I now tried this with Adelaine.

I said something like this: "Now feeling yourself in that place where your headaches started"—she nodded agreement—"now begin to *look* at your feet and *see* where they are and from your feet *look* out across the place and begin to *look* at all the things that are there and the peculiar relationship that they have and the way they are arranged in that special way."

Note again the visual words, but also note the other unspecified language and words that allow her to fill in the actual details of the memory. I then moved to auditory words.

"Now seeing all that you see and feeling all that you feel, now *listen*. *Listen* to the peculiar *sounds* of the place and the way you feel as you *listen*."

All of this took some time. I waited after each suggestion to be sure that her face and body appeared to be following my words. I was looking for a relaxed, fully attentive expression. She nodded agreement, which made it easier for me to know she was into the memory. After a few more moments, she spoke very softly and slowly, still breathing deeply and still with her face relaxed and un-furrowed. It was a remarkable experience to hear this nearly mute woman begin to talk and tell me her story.

In a weak and very slow voice, she told me a long story of her apartment and how she had moved there from Massachusetts a few months before. Her husband had died suddenly and she had moved to town to be near her only daughter and grandchild. She also had quit her job of many years. She told me that she was already in deep grief, and the move and the totally strange environment and culture change were overwhelming. Her withdrawal and sadness deepened. She spent most days in her gown, going nowhere, see-ing no one. Before her move, she had always worked. Now that was gone too. Except for her daughter, everything she had known and been accustomed to had vanished.

It was remarkable to sit and listen to a woman who had said virtually nothing become almost garrulous. Adelaine then told me the story of the onset of her headaches. As she mentioned the word "headache," her brow furrowed, her shoulders raised and tensed, and her breathing increased. She appeared to be in pain.

On that day in her apartment, she walked to the door of the refrigerator. As she reached for the handle, her bed shoes hit some water on the floor, causing her to slide headlong into a corner of a counter. She then fell backward, striking a sharp edge on the door-way. She was stunned and nearly unconscious. As she recovered her senses, she reached for the telephone, which had been knocked to the floor, and called her daughter. The daughter, hearing her mother in such distress, rushed over to the apartment and took her to the emergency room of the hospital. There they found no injury but admitted her for observation overnight.

Since that time, Adelaine had developed repeated severe at-tacks of headaches. Each time she called her daughter. Each time the daughter would rush to her mother's apartment. For several episodes, the daughter would rush her mother to the hospital. She had stopped the ER visits but still responded to her mother's calls by going over to the apartment. It had become a well-established pattern. Mother gets headache. Mother calls. Daughter responds. It was almost Pavlovian.

I was astonished at the amount of information that Adelaine provided. It was like a dam bursting, all this rush of words when none had come before. I believe, but I am not certain, that my using the correct kinds of words permitted this to happen. I think I was quite careful to test visual and auditory words repeatedly before I tried kinesthetic ones. Only a camera and sound recorder would have verified this memory. This was my first case using the notions of representational systems and the power of attending to the choice of words as a method of assisting a patient to recall a memory. The results were so dramatic and the experience so exhilarating that I wanted to record it here. It was perhaps my most successful intervention in my odyssey.

With the historical information about the origins of Adelaine's headaches, I began to think about how this knowledge might assist her in removing the headaches or at least in ameliorating their severity. I had a long discussion with her daughter. She was married, worked in an office as a filing clerk, and had a teenage daughter, Adelaine's only grandchild. I was struck by the attentiveness of the daughter to Adelaine and thought there must be some way to put that strength to better use. It seemed to me that the daughter might even be reinforcing the pattern of her mother's headaches. I did not put it that way to her, however.

After I talked with the psychiatrist, we agreed to discharge Adelaine to her apartment. This occurred after several more days in the hospital and a series of discussions with the psychiatrist and the daughter. The psychiatrist was intrigued with the techniques I was trying to use and encouraged me to follow the patient to see what would come of my suggestion. By this time, I had developed a close working relationship with the psychiatrist as we shared notes about the Bandler and Grinder model.

Here is what I was thinking. I thought the pattern of headache, although initially caused by the severe blow, was now "learned," if you will, and reinforced by the daughter's solicitous behavior. It had become a kind of Pavlovian response in reverse. (I did not go into any of this detail of thought with the daughter or Adelaine. I am doing it here so you will follow my line of thinking and my recommendations.) I thought if the daughter would completely change her behavior, the old behavior of the mother would vanish. There is a dictum in behavior modification that says ignored behavior will extinguish and disappear.

Here is what I suggested. I told the daughter that she must always answer the phone when her mother called. If the mother complained of a headache, the daughter must be very brief and say only a few lines and then hang up. She was to say the following lines: "Mother, I am so sorry you have a headache. I wish you did not. I will wait to see you when you feel better. I do not want to worry you with a visit when you are feeling so bad. The doctor says we should not talk on the phone when you are hurting. I will call you later." She was then to hang up as quickly as possible.

On the other hand, if her mother called and did not complain of a headache, the daughter was to rush over to her mother's apartment and visit, or if that was not possible, she was to talk for a long period on the phone, drawing her mother into many topics that she liked to talk about—every topic, that is, except headaches.

The daughter was quite perceptive and readily agreed to the trial. She was obviously tired of the calls from her mother and had begun to develop an understandable resentment of the degree of intrusion of her mother into her own life. She liked the idea.

The results came rapidly. Within a few weeks, the calls from the mother dropped from daily to a few per week. She continued to mention the headaches for the first several calls; then she dropped the subject entirely. The daughter had rushed over the first time her mother called with no mention of the headache; thereafter she just talked on the phone when her mother did not mention them. I talked on the phone with the daughter several times but never saw her again. I continued to see Adelaine for several years. We dealt mostly with her diabetes. She never mentioned the headaches again, and I did not ask her about them. I really do not know if the headaches went away or if Adelaine just quit talking about them. Either result was acceptable to me and, I can assure you, also to the daughter.

• • •

In many ways, my work with Adelaine was one of my most memorable cases. I do not think I have ever done a better job, before or since. There is a sense of deep satisfaction all the way through. Not only was I able to decode what she was trying to say but couldn't, but I did it with what I consider an elegant technique. And it is one I hope I have described in enough detail so that others can test it. The combined successes of trying a new method to elicit a most difficult history for the first time, having it work so well, and, for the same patient, developing a plan of action that relied on people other than the patient herself—also for the first time—and having it work equally well were tremendously rewarding experiences for me.

# 16
# The Woman Who Could Not Tell Her Husband Anything

When I first saw Joyce in the hospital, she was in coma from diabetic ketoacidosis. The scene was familiar. The cardiac monitors were running. Paper flowcharts were all over the bed table and the end of the bed. There were scattered blood-tinged syringes and empty blood-specimen tubes mixed among them. Long strips of EKG paper were becoming matted into the accumulated debris on the floor around the bed. Two nurses were taking a sample of urine for glucose testing from the Foley catheter tubing that ran from Joyce's urinary bladder. A resident and two interns were huddled over the bedside table looking at one of the flow sheets. Joyce lay unconscious, oblivious to the deliberate rush and hubbub that surrounded her.

She was breathing in the classic Kussmaul manner, very deep and regular and rapid breaths. I watched the body's miraculous compensation for acidosis—the blowing off of carbon dioxide to rid the body of its most soluble and effervescent acid, carbonic acid (derived from a mixture of carbon dioxide and water). Joyce's lungs were doing their job, responding to an incredibly complex feedback system. The insulin, along with the salt and water replacement, would allow her to do the rest. These cases are always touch and go. I have always thoroughly liked manipulating the biochemistry of the event. It takes a lot of knowledge of physiology and biochemistry to go through the full and proper treatment of a patient in diabetic ketoacidosis. The disease is a biochemically oriented internist's dream of the "good case." I suppose it is the medical equivalent of the repair of a ruptured heart to a chest surgeon.

I had not been called to see Joyce to care for her diabetes but to try to unravel why she was being admitted in coma almost every month. She had been in the hospital seven times in the past ten months, each time unconscious and in ketoacidosis from uncontrolled diabetes mellitus. There is a dictum I have found useful in such cases. It goes like this: "Recurrent diabetic ketoacidosis in a patient with childhood onset diabetes is usually due to the patient's not taking insulin." I did not make up the rule but heard it somewhere along the way in the blurred dozens of talks and articles I have heard or read about diabetic coma. If this rule applied in Joyce's case, we would have to arrive there by excluding all known medically treatable causes of diabetic ketoacidosis. It never works to pursue directly the possibility that someone stopped taking insulin on purpose to go into diabetic acidosis. Even raising the question with the patient builds resentment and resistance. The list of other known causes is quite long and includes a number of infectious diseases. All had already been either tested for or ruled out on previous admissions.

After I looked over Joyce's chart and checked what was being done, I called her private physician, an internist, to get his thoughts about the case. He had no clue why Joyce had such frequent and severe recurrences of acidosis. Extensive and exhaustive workups for the known precipitating causes had been negative on all prior admissions. He talked a bit about his feelings of failure for not keeping Joyce out of trouble.

There is a belief common among some internists that they are responsible for the total health of their patients in a very direct way, even when the patient is at home. This comes from the strict training in hospitals, where indeed the physician bears a heavy responsibility for the health and treatment of the hospitalized patient. This sense of responsibility often carries over into the outside world. Joyce's internist felt he was somehow at fault because Joyce kept returning with diabetic ketoacidosis, a condition ordinarily thought of as preventable. All his efforts to keep her out of trouble had failed.

I knew and shared his thoughts and feelings. You may recall Amy in Chapter 2. She was the young girl at Fort Hood, Texas, who had unregulated diabetes that became well regulated when a little girl and a kitten showed up on the scene. I wondered briefly, but without saying it to Joyce's internist, "What little girl or kitten is missing from Joyce's life?"

I had to wait until Joyce came out of coma to talk with her. By late afternoon, when I returned to see her, she was talking and taking liquids by mouth. I never fail to get some equivalent of goose bumps every time I witness a completely unconscious patient recover from diabetic coma and begin to talk as though nothing had happened. I had the same feelings when I spoke briefly with Joyce and told her of my reasons for seeing her. Her internist had asked me to see her to try to find out why she had so many episodes of coma.

The first words out of her mouth were interesting and revealing. She asked, "Well, are you a psychiatrist?" I had my first clue.

I said that I was not a psychiatrist. I asked if she thought she needed one. She shook her head and looked out the window. Her eyes watered and turned red. She bit inward on both lips and quickly shook her head again. I changed the subject, thinking she was about to cry. I had found that many patients in hospitals are on the verge of crying almost all the time. Some people have said that hospitals are grieving institutions, and that the number of patients with hidden depression or unresolved grief is very large, even as high as 20 percent. My own experience bears out that notion, and it was reaffirmed by Joyce's suppression of her tears.

• ◆ •

I had come to believe, contrary to a common contemporary notion, that facilitating a patient to cry is not helpful. In fact, it can be counterproductive. I had learned to detect at their earliest stages grief or sadness or whatever other internal states can cause tears. There is a dictum that says that for "every internal emotional state there is a full and visible external representation of that state, if you have the eyes and ears to detect it" (Bandler and Grinder 1982). What this means to me is that subtle changes in skin color, moisture content of the eyes, movements of the mouth, and the shape of eyes all reflect the internal emotional state of the patient—in Joyce's case, grief or sadness

I had also discovered that these external signs of internal emotional states occur several moments before they come into the full consciousness of the patient. If I distracted the patient, the signs of near crying quickly changed to the distracted state. As best I can tell, people, for a brief moment, are often not aware that they are about to cry. I tested this in one patient whom I had known and trusted for a long time, and he said he was not aware of any sadness or grief even though I had seen his eyes get quite red and watery and his lower lip quiver before I distracted him. I believe there is a considerable delay in most patients between the time external signs are visible and the onset of conscious awareness of internal feelings. (This notion could be tested more objectively with a properly designed set of experiments.) I used the phenomenon to follow patients along without putting them through another recall of a repeatedly painful memory.

I am not aware of any scientific foundation for the therapeutic value of getting someone to express emotions or feelings in a medical interview. In addition, I see no plausible benefit in having someone repeat a painful memory. It seems to me that it would only reinforce the original painful learning and make it even less accessible to moderation or removal. The goal should be removal or modification of the previously painful experience so that it is no longer painful. (There are methods to modify painful memories, but those are beyond the scope of this book.)

I do not mean by any of this that emotions of the moment

should go unexpressed. Actually, I do not know whether expressing them is good or bad. I just do not want to confuse the two states. Having someone recall a painful emotional experience is quite different from having a painful emotional experience in the present. My point is that I do not know with any certainty if it is helpful to get people to recall past painful memories. I know that the concept of ventilation of feelings is widely accepted as a helpful process. My plea is that such notions be tested with well-designed experiments. Whatever the truth is, I noted but usually distracted painful emotional states in most situations of recall.

• • •

I quickly distracted Joyce with some irrelevant questions and watched the redness in her eyes vanish. I told her I would return the next day and have a long talk with her. I left her with an injunction that I wanted her to think about overnight. Injunctions immediately before a departure from a room can be useful devices: Leave the patient with the most telling and searching question possible.

I said my favorite injunction very slowly and watched Joyce's face to be sure I held her attention; maintaining the attention of the patient is critical to any injunction. "All of us do things that we should not do, and we do not do those things that we should. I wonder if there is any possibility that you are doing something in either category. I wonder if you are doing something that you should not be doing. I can't imagine what that would be. I also wonder if there is something that you should be doing that you are not doing. I can't imagine what that would be either."

She nodded her head affirmatively to both statements but said, "No, there is nothing like that. I can't think of anything like that at all. I'm not at all sure what you are talking about." Her words were clipped.

Her positive nonverbal head-nodding responses and her negative verbal response are called "incongruence." I do not know the full significance of incongruence. I have assumed a working hypothesis that at the least, incongruence signifies a conflict of thoughts. Part of Joyce's mind understood and accepted my injunction. Another part did not.

It takes considerable experience and focused observation to detect incongruence. It is one of the findings I would most like to see tested with audiovisual recordings. Most of us, I suspect, miss incongruent responses. A clue to their presence in any encounter is when another person's response is confusing or irritating or seems inappropriate for the interchange. An incongruent response is not the only cause for these reactions, but it is a common one.

I responded to Joyce's nonverbal response. I said that even though neither she nor I knew the whole answer at that moment, I was sure of one thing.

"What's that?" she asked quickly.

"Your mind knows the answer." I left the room.

I saw Joyce daily for several days. Her physician was adjusting her diet and insulin dose to the levels that would allow her to go home. I held back from discussing anything other than trivial topics or questions about where she lived, what she did with her time, and what her husband did for his work—anything to allow her to bring up more meaningful topics. On the third day, she started to discuss her husband in some detail.

The picture I obtained was of a young man in his midtwenties who worked on the family farm with his father and two brothers. Joyce and her husband lived next door to his father. Her husband got up at dawn and worked until dark, came home, ate supper, fell asleep in front of the television set, and later got up and went to bed, only to repeat the cycle the next day and every other day but Sunday. On Sunday, they went to church and then spent the day next door with his family and all his nieces and nephews and brothers and sisters.

Joyce's most telling remark was, "He never listens to me. I can't get him to talk to me." I noted the auditory verbs.

I met the husband and had a long discussion with him about why he thought his wife was in the hospital so frequently. He had no idea and was puzzled. He was very worried and concerned and obviously cared a lot for his wife. And he also was oblivious to her needs for someone with whom to talk and someone who would listen.

In the course of my talks with him, it became apparent that he was a "show me" kind of person. He said things like, "If it don't look broke, then it ain't broke." He even said his wife went along looking well and healthy to him and then all of a sudden she "looked near death." He had the impression that Joyce got sick suddenly, but Joyce said she got sick over several days. It now became apparent to me that Joyce was predominantly an auditory person, while her husband was highly visual, at least in the way they preferred to process information. The verbs were heavily auditory for Joyce and nearly exclusively visual for the husband.

Proceeding on this assumption, I taught Joyce the notion that her husband did not understand words that spoke of sounds or talking as well as he understood words that used pictures or visual images. Instead of asking him to listen to her, which she had been doing, I suggested she ask him to look at her. Say, "I want you to *see* me. To *look* at me. I want you to *see* how I am doing. I want you to *see* what I am saying." Even, "Do you *see* what I mean?" I was explicit in teaching her the notion of his mind being tied to visual images and hers more to words and sounds.

The whole idea rang true. The husband said, "Well, I never knew she wanted me just to tell her I love her. All I do all day long is try to show her how much I do. Can't she see that I do love her?"

I tried to explain to him the concept that she needed to hear that he did, but I was unable to get his full attention. I decided to focus all my efforts on teaching Joyce, who by then showed interest in trying out the notion.

After her discharge from the hospital, I never saw Joyce or her husband again. Her physician, however, kept me posted on her progress. She had no admission for diabetic ketoacidosis or coma over the several years that followed. Within two years, she had her first pregnancy and produced a normal baby boy. Her diabetic control during pregnancy apparently had been excellent.

I asked her internist what he thought accounted for Joyce's turnaround. He said that Joyce had taught her husband to do her urine sugar tests so he could *see* how she was doing. (Home glucose monitoring was a technique still in the future.) Also she had taught him to draw up her insulin so he would *see* how much insulin she was taking. She also got him to *watch* her inject the insulin.

I do not know with certainty what stopped Joyce's frequent admissions for ketoacidosis. I want to believe that the instructions I gave allowed her to build a relationship with her husband founded on something other than having to go into ketoacidosis to get his attention and show him how sick she was. I never asked her if she stopped her insulin injections to produce ketoacidosis. I did not need to. She most likely had done just that.

I find it much more satisfying to leave that kind of truly embarrassing thing unsaid. Also I find it more productive to go for root causes whenever possible and make adjustments there rather than confront the more superficial causes. The omission of insulin was only a mechanism for something at a more profound level of organization. My model for this approach to Joyce was my notion that she and her husband had opposite brain processes and that they were not communicating. Joyce was auditory and did not see her husband's caring. Her husband was visual and did not hear his wife's distress until he could literally see her near death. If that were the case, then correction of that process would have a much more pervasive beneficial effect than merely attacking the cessation of insulin injections.

♦ ♦ ♦

I will never know what turned Joyce around. My representation that a correction of communication between Joyce and her husband based on the model of visual and auditory ways of communicating may or may not be correct. Only repeated observations with other patients would confirm or refute the model. Again, these ideas call out for well-designed studies and experiments to test the notions of auditory or visual speech in other patients. I report the case here because the turnaround was so definite and dramatic. The only therapy or treatment offered were instructions to Joyce on how to get her husband's attention without going into diabetic ketoacidosis. It seemed to work.

# 17
# Staying Out of God's Way

Marie was sixteen years old, an upcoming junior in high school. Until she got sick, she was head majorette for the marching band.

She had two older brothers and a younger sister. All four had been highly successful in their school activities and academic performances. Both the mother and father were in high school education. The father was a high school principal, and the mother taught library science. The family lived in a nearby state and had been referred to me because of Marie's long and debilitating illness. By this time, I had gained a reputation of taking on tough cases. Marie would turn out to be one of my most difficult. She had not walked in more than a year and was paralyzed in both legs.

To say simply that Marie was cheerful would be a major understatement. She bubbled with cheerfulness and happiness even when she discussed her paralysis. She might as well have been telling you about a comedy. She never stopped smiling broadly. Nothing got her down. She gave the appearance of being on top of the world. To my notion, her outward behavior was inappropriate for the gravity of her situation. It has been called *la belle indifference* and usually is associated with patients who are labeled hysterical.

"Hysterical" in this use of the word is usually associated with what are called conversion symptoms. "Conversion" means that the symptoms cannot be explained on the basis of objective physiological abnormalities or by the presence of physical disease. While the term is old and descriptive, it dictates no specific therapy or approach. It certainly is no help to tell a patient that she or he is hysterical. It is the kind of label I keep in the back of my mind. I do not let the term get in the way of approaching the patient in a direct and honest manner based on what I see and hear with my own eyes and ears. I try to disregard the label when I am encountering the patients or their families. I find that if I approach the patient as if the diagnosis is unknown, I do better in outlining a helpful strategy. That is the manner in which I tried to approach Marie and her family.

I spent the first several outpatient visits going over data from earlier doctors and hospital admissions. The history was very complicated, and I do not want to bore you with all the details. It is, however, essential to give you enough information so that you can follow the case and my clinical reasoning.

Marie had "never been sick a day in her life" until about a year and a half before I saw her. The first sign of her illness was a high fever and severe muscle aches, particularly in her calf muscles. The fever lasted more than two weeks. She also developed some enlarged lymph nodes in her neck and a low-grade sore throat. The indirect test (all that was available at that time) for mononucleosis was positive, and a diagnosis of infectious mononucleosis was made. She had the typical blood-smear findings of atypical lymphocytes, which reverted to normal within a month. I had no reason to quarrel with the diagnosis as correct at the time it was made. The only problem was that Marie did not get well. In fact, she gradually got worse.

Let me clarify here. Marie had what looked like and tested like infectious mononucleosis. There was no argument on that point. All the tests returned to normal and the fever disappeared. It therefore was assumed that she had infectious mononucleosis and that she would get well symptomatically. She did the opposite and got worse. She became paralyzed in both legs the month after the fever.

Marie had seen a number of specialists and had been admitted on three occasions to other hospitals. The number and variety of tests and diagnostic procedures were legion. They included three separate spinal taps, a myelogram of the spine, electromyograms, a nerve biopsy, and a muscle biopsy from the calf. All the results were normal. Using my most vivid imagination, I could not think of a single test that had not been done that would fit the case. I ordered some repeat blood tests to reaffirm their negativity and waited.

Marie had received a variety of diagnoses before I saw her. On one occasion early in her paralysis, she was told she had disseminated histoplasmosis, a deep fungus infection that acts like disseminated tuberculosis and is associated with multiple small nodules in both lungs. To confuse the issue, she had a positive skin test for histoplasmosis, but so do many people in the general population in the area of the country where she lived. The positive skin test meant only that she had been exposed to the fungus in her tissues. It did not mean active disease, either past or present. There was nothing about her clinical history that remotely acted like disseminated histoplasmosis.

Marie also had been told she had a "myositis." This nonspecific term for inflamation of muscle is useless. A muscle biopsy had been done and overread as diseased. A review of the slides by several pathologists, at my request, confirmed that the muscle tissue seen on biopsy was indeed normal. In cases like Marie's, there are always confusing and conflicting pieces of clinical evidence to cloud and confound the problem. "Myositis" is often a weak diagnosis and a term used far too loosely. Marie did not have myositis of any sort.

Finally, on her third admission she was told the whole thing was in her head and that she needed a psychiatrist. In fact, her mother's opening comment to me was, "Don't tell me that Marie needs a psychiatrist. We don't need you to tell us that because we have already been told that. We need you to help us get Marie well. If there ever was a normal and well-adjusted young girl, it is Marie. She is not insane."

Marie's mother was extremely upset by the earlier suggestion that her daughter needed psychiatric care and made it clear to me that they resented the doctor's saying that. Her response to the suggestion that "the problem is in your head" is nearly universal. I will say it once more: I have never seen that statement help. Yet I hear over and over from many patients that some doctor told them it was all in their head. It is a sure way to remove a patient from a practice. Maybe that is the intention of those who use it.

I had my work cut out if I accepted Marie and her mother for care. The father was a remote, nearly ghostlike figure in the whole episode of care. I was at the peak of my interest in difficult patients and frankly, Marie's problem was irresistible. I had no idea how I would proceed when I told them I would give it a try. I did say that if I had not helped in three months they should fire me and move to another physician. As I think about the case now, that statement may have been more determinative than anything else I said. Its hidden message was, "You have only three months to get well."

I spent an inordinate amount of time reading the reports from the other hospitals and doctors in the presence of Marie, her mother and father, and anyone else in the family. I read them slowly and asked for amplification of the facts. I read aloud all the technical and medical terms and explained them if anyone had questions. I saw Marie for four visits before I arrived at any conclusion or suggestion. I was laying out my facts for the diseases Marie did not have. I did not know what she had . . . *yet.*

Several findings were especially important in my arriving at a plan of action. First and most important, I found Marie's neurological examination to be entirely within normal limits. She had all deep-tendon reflexes intact. I did what I call my most extensive neurological examination and found no defect except that Marie could not walk normally when instructed to do so. She would attempt to stand if I held her. When I let go, she wobbled in a kind of ducklike gait and then she crossed her legs and attempted to walk with her legs crossed. She then slammed into the wall of the hallway and bounced off it into the wall on the other side, where she slid onto the floor into a crumpled and extraordinarily awkward position. Both hands were pinned behind her hips. Remarkably, she made no effort to withdraw her arms but lay there as if now her arms were paralyzed too. The whole exercise was grossly distorted and exaggerated. Her gait and performance were typical of either malingering or of the conversion type of hysterical paralysis.

An analysis of her gait showed that it took very great strength to reproduce what she had done. To be able to duck walk and then to walk with both legs crossed and at the same time maintain balance takes a lot of muscle power.

One other finding of note was the striking difference in strength between what she could do in the official muscle examination and what she could do when attempting to stand or walk. She showed almost no motion when officially asked to move her legs, yet she could do all that I have described when held up and told to try to walk. This discrepancy is also characteristic of conversion paralysis or malingering. By any definition, Marie would be called a patient with conversion reaction or conversion hysterical paralysis.

I now had to figure out how to deal with both Marie and her mother. Emotionally they seemed inseparable. I knew that a direct psychological or psychiatric approach would not only fail but also be rejected. It had been tried and failed. There was no demonstrable medical disease to label and treat. Whatever I came up with would have to be entirely believable to everyone concerned. The time to take action had come. There were no more tests to do.

I had learned that whatever fails once will continue to fail. If a clinical approach does not work the first time, it will not work the second or third or whatever number of times you try it. Some clinicians seem to think that if a psychological approach has failed for a previous physician, all they have to do is present the suggestion more emphatically or more logically, and it will take. They seem to have difficulty believing that logic will not always win out. Just because the clinical evidence may be convincing for a diagnosis does not mean that the patient will accept the diagnosis or the treatment. I recalled Sweet Thing and her hypoglycemia from unneeded insulin and the mistake I made on insisting on removing the diagnosis of diabetes. I would not make that same mistake with Marie.

Marie's family was religious in the most fundamental way. They frequently told me that only God could really cure and that with their strong faith, they believed that God would cure Marie. It was plain to me that whatever I suggested had to fit their strong religious beliefs also.

Here is what I did and the reasoning I used. I told Marie and her mother that Marie had a serious disease a year and a half ago. As I said this, I paid very close attention to their facial expressions, looking for what I have come to recognize as the look of undivided attention. The face shifts into a blank expression, squint lines vanish, the mouth droops. With full attention, some people slowly nod in agreement. This is clearly a mild form of trance. If the attention shifts, there is no point in going on. It is essential to maintain full attention. Without it, nothing will be accomplished. It is what I came to call "full rapport."

Continuing very slowly, I said that I was not sure what the disease was but that whatever it was, it had been very severe and very, very serious. Marie was lucky to be alive. I went on to explain that I had spent most of my time testing to see if there was evidence of any residual of the disease. Despite all my efforts, I could find no evidence for any remaining active disease. Whatever this disease was, it was now gone.

However, I had found considerable aftereffects of the disease, which had taken a toll on Marie's body, especially on her legs, which had been rendered very weak—close to but not actually paralyzed.

All in all, I declared her in a state of convalescence or recovery. I thanked them for coming to see me and making me look like such a good doctor. I explained that if they had not come to see me, Marie had been about to get well anyway. This way, it would make me look like an extraordinary doctor and even appear that I had cured her, when both they and I knew that things did not work that way. (I left plenty of room for whatever religious belief they wanted to apply.) Now, I said, I did think there was some urgency for Marie to go ahead and get well ahead of time.

Here, I have to digress and boast a bit. My choice of the phrase "get well ahead of time" may be my all-time best injunction to a patient. When I said it, I slowed my words and lowered my pitch. I wanted her mind to hear "*Get well*."

In fact, I explained, there was some danger and risk in not going ahead and getting well ahead of schedule. I described how muscles that lie unused will atrophy and become useless. I used the analogy of the atrophy that we see when a cast is removed from an arm (her brother had a broken arm a few years back, and I reminded their memory of the atrophy of his arm when it came out of the cast). I told them that there is always a critical time window for convalescence, and if the time window passes, there could be permanent and irreversible damage to the muscles.

I suggested that Marie be admitted to the hospital for intensive physical therapy so that the critical time window would not pass and leave the muscles permanently weak. In this way, Marie could speed up her convalescence. Both Marie and her mother had nodded agreement to everything I said. I had maintained their full rapt attention throughout my talk. I admitted Marie the next day.

Before her admission, I visited the physical therapy department and explained the situation to the therapists. I asked that only one therapist be assigned to Marie. Marie was to come to the center twice daily for vigorous workouts.

For the first three days, Marie's room was filled with her high school classmates and friends. The whole thing had turned into a circus, and Marie was no better, although she stayed all smiles as she told me that she was actually getting worse. I called in her mother and father and we had a conference in front of Marie.

I told them they had taken what I said about a critical time window far too lightly. I did not know if the window was three months or two months or just two weeks. I had somehow not conveyed the urgency of the time factor. I emphasized *"two weeks,"* and it was the last time interval I said. (If you give a patient a list of symptoms, he or she will be most likely to choose the last one mentioned. I hoped for the same phenomenon here.)

I wanted all friends prohibited from visiting. I wanted the phone removed from Marie's room. I wanted all family to limit visits to evenings only. I wanted Marie to go to physical therapy twice a day, take naps, do no reading, watch no television, and make no phone calls. She was to convalesce in quiet and peace if she was to get well "ahead of schedule."

By this time, Marie had begun to argue with me that she would get well ahead of schedule and still see her friends and use the phone. I insisted on removing all contact with her friends and limiting family contact. Her mother and father readily agreed and told Marie to do what I said. Marie was fuming.

The next day, they called me to physical therapy and told me that Marie had actually walked a few steps. I said that was just a fluke and did not mean anything and left immediately, waving at Marie without talking to her.

Each day, Marie showed additional progress. Each day, I was "unimpressed" and pooh-poohed the significance of it. On the fifth day, Marie stood in one corner of the physical therapy room and suddenly began to turn cartwheels across the mat. I smiled and nodded and walked up to her.

"Well, I was wrong again. I thought you were just fooling me with your improvements, when you really were getting better all along. I just couldn't believe you were getting well that fast. Are you ready to go home?"

Marie nodded and smiled even broader than ever, if that was possible. The whole family came that afternoon to take her home.

I had stated everything in very nonspecific language. None of my terms had carried specific meanings, yet all sounded like I was being very specific. What does "getting well ahead of time" really mean? What does "convalescent phase" really mean? I said that "the illness had gone." I said it had left her muscles weak (that was obvious). I stated everything in a way that was plausible and in a way that could not be directly refuted. I paced the mother's belief and used it to formulate a plan that was acceptable to her and Marie. All I did was create a way out for Marie. The only action I really took was to withdraw her from all friends and from all entertainment. I removed all secondary gain from her paralysis. She had to get well to be with her friends, and she did.

Marie's mother called me aside. She went into a long discussion of how thankful she was that Marie was healed. She expressed a sincere belief that God had healed her and that I had not got in the way of God in the manner those other doctors had. She thanked me for not getting in God's way.

I thought to myself that hers might be one of the highest compliments I had ever received, even though I would not have thought of it in the same terms. Maybe she was right. Maybe at our best, we doctors do stay out of God's way.

# 18

# A Paradoxical Approach

Ordinary and standard clinical approaches fail with some patients. In the patient I am now going to discuss—I will call her Regina— some will say that I went too far or that I should not have done what I did.

I first saw Regina in the hospital. She was under the care of an orthopedist. Regina had no disease except severe and intractable back pain. The orthopedist knew of my interest in difficult patients and asked me to see her to find out if I had anything to suggest. Regina's lab work and physical exam were within normal limits. All the x-ray and myelographic studies of her spinal cord, nerve roots, and bony spine were also normal. She had undergone three back operations, none of which had helped in the least.

Regina looked and acted angry most of the time. She spoke in a shrill loud voice and made exasperated expressions and sighs in response to most questions. She would not look at me but looked at the ceiling most of the time or down at the bedcovers, which she fiddled with a lot. She looked tired and had dark circles under her eyes and a mouth that drooped when she was not talking. She delighted in telling me about her past medical and surgical failures.

I asked one of my favorite questions. "How long have you been in bad health?" (Sometimes I phrased it, "When were you last in really good, robust health?") She answered that she had been sick as long as she could remember. Sometime in her first year of life, she had a protracted encounter with a physician who told her mother that Regina was "sickly and underdeveloped." Regina's mother told her that she would never be a well person.

Regina got married at age fifteen (against her mother's advice), ran away from home for three months, then returned to live with her mother and father along with her husband and, in a short time, a baby boy. Regina was now thirty-two years old. She, her husband, and their sixteen-year-old son still lived in the family home with Regina's mother and father. Regina's husband, Floyd, worked at a local dairy farm and was rarely home except to sleep.

Regina spent more than an hour recounting all her unhappy encounters with the medical profession. Rather than skirt over these, I drew her out on each case, asking who the doctor was, what medicine had been prescribed, and what surgery was performed. I asked her to tell me in great detail all the side or toxic effects of each drug and every complication she had with each operation.

She was smiling and sometimes laughing as she told me of one bad outcome after another. She said she was allergic to or had become nauseated on every known pain medication. I spent several minutes getting her to name every drug she could not take—Demerol, morphine, Dilaudid, codeine, aspirin, phenacetin, caffeine, APCs, Doane's back-pain pills, and more than a dozen sleeping pills and tranquilizers. She knew them all by name and dosage and told me what each one did that was bad for her—skin rashes, headaches, nausea, constipation, burning lips, itching legs, watering eyes, ringing ears, and many more symptoms that the pills that were supposed to help her had caused.

Then she went into all the complications surgery had produced. After the first back operation, she could not walk for three months and then only with a cane. She developed a rash from lying in bed that took six months to heal. These complications were compounded by many of the drug reactions she had just listed.

Between the first and second back operations, she had a miscarriage and had to have a D and C (dilation and curettage) to stop the bleeding she had discovered in the middle of the night; she said she was "nearly bleeding to death before they got me to the hospital." She developed a bladder infection after the D and C and then an allergic reaction to the antibiotic, for which she took cortisone, which caused her to swell "all over."

After the second back operation, she had severe abdominal pains, which led to an exploratory abdominal operation, following which she could not take food by mouth for three weeks. She was so weak after the second back operation that her husband had to carry her in his arms around the house and to the bathroom. The third back operation had been a year before I saw her, and the numbness in both feet that followed that operation had just cleared up a few months ago.

She told all of this and much more as fast as I could listen. I would interrupt her to amplify details for each story and each complication or drug reaction. I wanted her to go into as much detail as possible about each problem. I wanted her to know I had heard every word she said.

I left after the first visit, saying that I had a lot of things to think about and that I did not know what I would recommend. I had no idea at the time what to tell her.

About this time in my search for new ways to deal with difficult patients like Regina, I had read a book called *Change* (Watzlawick, Weakland, and Fisch 1974) The authors described a patient very much like Regina who they posited liked to defeat experts. They mentioned a class of people who, for whatever reason, play a game of defeating experts. There is only one way that an expert (a clinician, in this case) can be defeated and help the patient at the same time, the authors suggest: a therapeutic paradox.

According to the method described in *Change*, the patient (in this case, Regina) is saying unconsciously: "No matter what you do, I will stay sick. You have heard all my old experiences with doctors, and in each one I did not get well. In fact, no matter what the doctor did, I got worse. Every operation and medicine made me get sicker." Of course, Regina did not say this out loud, but it was clearly her message. The therapeutic paradox the authors suggested is what I tried with Regina.

I discussed the case with the orthopedist and he agreed with the approach I outlined. He had nothing to offer the patient and could think of no other tests or operations that would help. She had been in physical therapy for months with no help; in fact, she thought she had strained her back even further with some of the treatments.

The next day, I sat down by Regina's bed with my notes in hand. I asked the head nurse on the unit to be there and witness what I told Regina. I was very anxious because I had never been as frank as I intended to be with Regina, and I could not predict what reaction she might have. I intended to tell her exactly what I thought about her present condition and what I thought would happen to her in the future. I was going to follow the rules of the paradox, because I believed it was as close to the truth as I could get. If it helped Regina, fine. If it did not, I could not imagine how it would hurt her except to make her angry.

I recounted in great and slow detail all her previous operations and the complications and problems she had after each one. She nodded in full agreement to each of my retellings of her accounts. I even asked her to interrupt me if I left out any important detail. I soon had her rapt attention. After I went over all the operations, I went on to the drugs and retold the side effects and toxic reactions she had told me about. I listed each one separately. I named all her previous doctors and what she said they had told her and how she thought each one was wrong and how each one had not helped but had indeed made her worse. She nodded again and again. I do not recall ever having anyone's full and undivided attention to the degree I now had Regina's. She was hanging on every word I said. Her face was blank of any expression and her mouth was slightly open.

I then went back over the physician list, naming each doctor who had seen her and what problems he or she had caused. And then I said something like this: "I know some of these doctors, and they are fine physicians and surgeons. I am sure the others are too. Why, I wonder to myself, do you think I would be any better than those you have seen. I probably am no better than those doctors, yet you come to me and Dr. S. [the orthopedist] and think we can help you when all these others have failed."

Regina started to speak, but I interrupted her. This is what I think I told her next. "You have had some of the best medical and surgical treatments, and it has not helped you. You have seen some of the best doctors. You have had every test known to medical science. You are allergic to or you get sick with every known pain-relieving drug. There are no other tests, no other operations, no other drugs to recommend. I don't know of any more doctors to recommend either. You appear to me to be beyond medical science."

Here, I started the paradox. "I have known a lot of patients like you, and I wish I had told them what I am about to tell you. In my professional opinion, you will never get better. You will stay sick the rest of your life. You will probably have a lot more operations and complications and bad effects. I am sure you will take a lot more drugs and get allergic or have side effects with each one. The older you get, the sicker you will get. I wish I had something, anything, positive to suggest but I don't. I don't know of anything at all to suggest or recommend. And I don't know, nor have I read of, any doctor who I think might be able to help you. In my opinion, you are simply beyond medical science."

She was flushed in the face and appeared very angry. She breathed between her clenched teeth very fast. Her lower jaw jutted forward. Her fists were clenched. Her eyebrows were lowered. I thought, "Now I have really done it." I stayed calm and sat there with as little expression as I could muster. I knew I was right, and I believed what I said. I would take what came.

Regina stared at me. "You mean to tell me you are not going

to treat me? Well then, maybe you just better send me to some to other doctor."

I explained that maybe she did not understand what I had said to her. I told her again slowly and calmly that I did not know of any doctors that could help her.

She went into a tirade about doctors in general and me in particular. She could not wait to call her husband and tell him what I had told her. She could not believe the "way I had treated her." I stood and said that I would be available to tell her husband the same thing I had told her. I suggested we go ahead and discharge her that afternoon, since there was nothing more we could do for her. I asked the nurse to call me when Regina's husband got there so I could repeat what I had said to him.

I felt drained. It had taken all my courage to sit there and tell the patient all that I had said. I was very careful to say exactly what I thought and what I could document. Every bit of what I said was what I believed. I had seen many patients like Regina, and they had indeed gone on to have many more operations and to get complications that might have been avoided. I had never seen a patient with the duration and intensity of symptoms Regina had get the slightest bit better. I had only told her what I thought.

In the back of my mind was the paradox of Watzlawick, Weakland, and Fisch and the hope that my directness and honesty might somehow win out. If indeed Regina was playing a game of defeating the expert, then I had certainly set her up to defeat me—but only by getting better. If she got worse, then *she* was defeated. If she went to another doctor, then *she* was defeated. If she took other medicines, then *she* was defeated. If she had another operation, then again *she* was defeated. The only way she could win, if the game concept was correct, was to get well. Of course, the entire notion of a game could be completely off base. If so, I had only been honest in telling Regina my somewhat unusual and heterodoxical thoughts.

Floyd was in the room when I came back that afternoon. He

was pacing the floor and turned to me when I entered. "What's this you told my wife about not believing she is sick? That she is faking the whole thing. That she is just making up her disease."

I asked him to sit down and called for the head nurse to be present. I asked the nurse to interrupt me if I said anything to the husband different from what I had told the patient in the morning. I then repeated as close to verbatim as I could what I had told Regina. I paced myself in the same slow manner and in the same detail about the drugs and surgery. I looked for Floyd's full attention and matched my talking speed to his facial expressions. He calmed down and listened intently. All the anger left his face. He began to nod when I told him that he must have spent a lot of money and a lot of time trying to get his wife well. I was simply saying that I did not think another doctor would help and that I did not know of anyone to suggest. Since she had taken all the pain medicines and none had helped and all of them had made her sick, then it only made sense that there were no medicines left to take. I asked, "Isn't it time just to quit?" I suggested that he take her home, since I had no other suggestions. I was sorry that I did not have any, but I did not.

He said almost nothing but appeared to be in deep thought. He stood when I left and said good bye.

I did not hear anything from or about Regina for more than six months. I did not expect ever to hear from her again. Then one day Floyd called me from a pay phone somewhere in Kansas. He told me a long and involved story of their life since they had left the hospital. First, he wanted to thank me for being the only doctor to be honest with them. Within a few weeks of leaving the hospital, they had moved to Kansas where he had found a better job. It was the first time they had ever lived away from Regina's parents' home. Regina had not seen a doctor and vowed to die before she would ever see another one. He went on to say that Regina spent a good bit of time berating me and saying what a sorry excuse for a doctor I was, how wrong I was, and how if it killed her she would stay healthy the rest of her life. He told me that Regina had a deep hate for me and that she would never forgive me for what I had said about her, how belittling I had been, and how much I had misjudged her character. He said he did not want Regina to know he had ever called me, but he did appreciate what I had told her and he understood what I had done.

I never saw Regina or her husband again and I never had the nerve to tell another patient what I told Regina, although I saw a lot more just like her. I kept thinking I would, but I never did.

# 19
# You Can't Be Everybody's Doctor

When I first saw Veronica, I was still working closely with Dr. Harry Abram, head of liaison psychiatry at Vanderbilt. My encounter with her occurred early in my experiences with patients who had symptoms of unknown origin. I have put her story toward the end because she is an extreme example of symptoms of unknown origins.

Veronica was twenty-six years old and was on the faculty of a nearby junior college nursing school. The dean of the nursing school had referred her to see me. Veronica was covered in bruises. Some looked superficial but others looked deep and purple—the kind I have always associated with third-stage clotting disorders or with leukemia. The superficial bruises were all paired in a butterfly pattern, a telltale sign that they are self-inflicted. Pinching the skin to the point of bruising always leaves a pair of bruises. The other giveaway in self-inflicted bruises is their complete absence between the shoulder blades, an area the person cannot reach.

This combination of superficial self-inflicted butterfly bruises and deeper ecchymoses (where blood has escaped into the tissues from ruptured blood vessels) characteristic of third-stage clotting disorders left me puzzled. However, the two types of bruises were not the only puzzling clinical features with Veronica.

She had grown up the only child of missionaries in Southeast Asia and told harrowing stories of one injury after another. As I was examining her eyes, she casually mentioned that her left eye had been sliced when a knife in her hand slipped. She said the vitreous ran down her cheek and she had to hold the eyeball in place with her hand until they got to the nearest village. She said the missionary doctor sewed the eye back in place. When I questioned the absence of a scar, she told me what a wonderful surgeon the doctor had been.

There was some dramatic story for nearly every organ I palpated or discussed. Her heart had been inflamed when she was a child. She had had a rare pulmonary lesion that finally had healed. She had vomited blood, had had blood in her stools and in her urine. She had been in shock from blood loss from a jeep accident in the jungles of Borneo. Both legs had been broken when she fell out of a tall tree. She told all these stories in a calm, nearly bored tone of voice.

I stopped passing comments and just listened to one story after another. I think I said something like, "It's a wonder you are still alive."

I admitted her to the hospital to work up her coagulation status. Admissions to hospitals were readily available in those days. They provided wonderful opportunities to observe and to get to know patients. Veronica's clotting time was greatly prolonged, as was her test that pointed toward a circulating anticoagulant. Both defects were corrected in the test tube with protamine sulfate, the agent known to reverse heparin's anticoagulating effect. To make a long story shorter, Veronica was obviously injecting herself with heparin, and she was also pinching herself to produce the smaller superficial bruises.

I called in my psychiatric associate, Harry Abram, to help. He and I had previously had long discussions about patients who inflict diseases on themselves—so-called factitious or factitial diseases. We had been waiting for the next such case to come along. He wanted to see if he could make any psychiatric sense out of the patient. At that time, and it still may be true, the literature contained no factitial patients who had been carefully observed or treated in psychiatry over a long period. Harry was interested in uncovering the psychodynamics of such patients.

After we had corrected the heparin effect in Veronica and all her clotting factors were back to normal, I discharged her from the hospital. We had a clear understanding that she was to see both me and Harry Abram in follow-up. I had been very direct in telling her that I knew of the heparin injections and warned her of the danger associated with her continuing them. She continued denying she had given herself these injections, even after discharge. I felt uncomfortable continuing to see her, but I had made a pact with Abram to follow one such patient with him—no matter what.

The next time I saw Veronica was about a month later. She had a huge abscess on her upper outer left arm, near the shoulder. She said she had been letting her student nurses practice injections on her, and obviously one of the students must have broken sterile technique. I called the dean of the nursing school and inquired about the student nurses using instructors' arms for practice sites. She called back to tell me that had not happened. Again, Veronica denied any self-infliction. I called Abram and suggested we end our pact. He insisted that he was beginning to make headway, despite the abscess occurrence. Once more, I reluctantly agreed to continue to follow Veronica medically.

Within a few weeks after the abscess had been drained, Veronica came into the emergency room, and the physician on call admitted her with a fever of 104 degrees. The next morning when I saw her, her temperature was 102 degrees with a pulse rate of 76 per minute. I called the nurse and we retook the temperature under observation. It was 98.8 degrees. Obviously, Veronica had heated the thermometer. Again, she denied it straight out, saying she had no explanation for the sudden drop in fever. Again I called Abram and he urged me to continue, saying something like, "Well, you didn't expect we would make quick progress on such a tough clinical problem, did you?"

Over the next two months, Abram saw Veronica weekly and reported to me that he was establishing strong rapport with her but still had no ideas of the psychodynamics or the origins of Veronica's need to self-inflict disease.

The next time I saw Veronica, she was complaining of extreme weakness. She was as pale as bedclothes. Her hematocrit was twenty-one, and I admitted her to the hospital. She showed signs of obvious blood loss with a rapid pulse. Her blood smears also showed evidence of iron deficiency. I began to transfuse her. She told me her menses had been extremely heavy and that was why she showed blood-loss anemia.

That afternoon when I entered Veronica's room, I found her running blood from the IV in her arm into the trash can by her bedside. She was continuing to bleed herself in the face of a severe anemia. That was it. I called Abram; we transferred Veronica to the psychiatric unit. When she was finally discharged, I gave her written notice that she must find another medical doctor, and I resigned from her care. Abram said he would continue to see her for psychiatric care.

Several months went by. Abram told me Veronica had stopped coming to see him. Several more months went by, and then I got a call from a hospital in Atlanta. Veronica has been admitted with severe anemia. She told the doctor there that I had been treating her for acute leukemia. I shared my failed experiences with him and wished him more luck than I had had in treating Veronica.

At that time in my practice, I was enjoying two of the most gripping fantasies young physicians can have—a sense of omnipotence and a belief that I could rescue every single patient in distress. Veronica's self-inflictions challenged both fantasies, a circumstance I found very difficult to accept. I did not see that the only language such patients have is self-infliction. I never learned to translate their language into one that I could understand and accept.

• • •

A long time ago, one of my professors wisely said, "You cannot be everybody's doctor. Pick and choose carefully." Every physician will have some patients who do not match. Balint is correct that apostolic functions predetermine the choices a physician has. My own apostolic functions preclude my taking on patients who persist in self-inflicted diseases. Veronica taught me that. To those physicians who can treat the Veronicas of this world, I can only say I wish you well. You are a rare breed, and I hope you will record your experiences for all to read.

# 20
# In Tune with the Patient

My journey didn't end with my adoption of Engel's biopsychosocial model as a clinical paradigm. I knew that I lacked the reflexes and clinical tools this broader clinical model would require. It was time for me to retool and learn to listen and to guide and coach patients. I had to undergo a "slight but significant change in my own personality," in Balint's terms (1957).

Armed with my experiences with Carl Rogers, Joseph Sapira, and the videotaping sessions in Fairhope, I found new methods of interviewing and intervening. These methods include:

- Having the primary intention of being maximally helpful with each patient.
- Honoring the personal integrity of each patient.
- Approaching the patient in a mild state of awe, to watch and wonder and listen.
- Making no distinction in level of interest between physical, social, psychological, or spiritual information.
- Avoiding cuing when asking questions about symptoms.
- Accepting the patient as having symptoms of unknown origin even at the initial visit.
- Learning to listen and reflect back what I hear until there is nodding agreement from the patient.

- Learning to gain and hold the full attention of the patient and, by watching the facial expressions, knowing when it is achieved.
- Paying attention to the breathing of the patient and sometimes matching my breathing to the rate and depth of the patient's breathing.
- Paying attention to the posture and body positions of the patient.
- Watching the face of the patient, paying attention to representations of emotion in the face and using those facial expressions as guides to the patient's attention, understanding, and internal emotional states.

I can lump all of these into what can be called "establishing full attention and rapport" with the patient. If these steps are blocked or not accepted by the patient, the encounters will become difficult, if not impossible. Such a reaction from the patient should strongly suggest that the patient is enjoying secondary gain from being sick.

The next steps, beyond establishing rapport, are directed at assisting the patient to discover or recollect what he or she is doing or not doing to produce the symptoms. I suggest this method be called physician-directed recollection (PDR).

These steps are:

- Avoiding specific diagnoses and disease labels until certain.
- Saying "I do not know what you have . . . *yet.*"
- Using unspecified language when asking questions.
- Embedding confronting-type questions in "I wonder if . . ." statements.
- Assisting the patient to find the pattern or variation of the symptoms.

- Having the patient use a diary when appropriate.
- Suggesting that the patient may be doing something he or she should not be doing or not doing something he or she should be doing.
- Continuing to delve into variables even when a medical disease is present.

In assisting the patient to uncover previously hidden correlations, I found it very helpful to pay attention to verbs in his or her speech. I found some patients to be either highly verbal or highly visual as expressed through visual or auditory verbs. I believe other patients operate more through feelings or kinesthetic systems. By switching my verbs to match the verbs of the patients, I was able to assist some of them to recover otherwise hidden associations that correlated with their symptoms. Milton Erickson and Carl Rogers exerted a heavy influence on my clinical approach. Both saw these approaches as entering the world of the patient. (see Erickson and Rossi 1979; Haley 1986, 1987; Rogers 1961.)

What were the outcomes of these procedures in those patients who had symptoms of a chronic nature and who had failed to have a diagnosis established after a reasonable medical workup? As I outlined in Chapter 9, each patient I saw with chronic symptoms of unknown origin fell into one of five categories.

## 1.  *The patient has a hidden or obscure medical disease that explains the symptoms.*

I want to emphasize that I am not talking about all patients with medical diseases. I am describing a subset of patients who have missed diagnoses of medical diseases that are producing their symptoms or problems. The medical diseases that fit into this category will usually be very rare diseases a clinician would not readily think of, or the symptoms will be unusual symptoms for a common disease. With these, as with all patients, careful guidance and diary keeping will often lead one to the underlying medical disease. Since I excluded all patients with documented diseases from my study series, I did not write very much about this category in the book. I did, however, see a number of such patients over the years.

The missed diseases I encountered included hypothyroidism. A spectacular example of this was Mrs. Johnson in Chapter 3, whose reclusive and demented state was reversed with thyroid hormone. I also saw patients with missed diagnoses of hyperthyroidism, hypopituitarism, all sorts of low-grade anemias, a variety of worm infestations (in returning Korean brides at Fort Hood), Cushing's syndrome, porphyrias, vitamin deficiencies (in bulimic patients), hypopotassemia, hyponatremia, hypercalcemia, and malnutrition from gastrointestinal malabsorption, among others. There is no need to make an exhaustive list. I only want to be sure to put medical diseases at the top of the list of categories for patients with symptoms of unknown origin:

*It is the first duty of a physician to miss no treatable medical disease.*

Sometimes combinations of factors produce the symptoms, even when the diagnosis of a medical disease is very clear. Tinsley Harrison, founding editor of *Harrison's Principles of Internal Medicine* (1950), was a master of teasing out symptoms of this sort. I attended his weekly conferences at the University of Alabama in Birmingham and recall the case of a man with documented angina pectoris. This was in the years before coronary surgery, and the goal then was to prescribe medications and a plan to allow each patient to lead as full and active a life as possible within the limitations of the coronary disease.

This man had most of his angina in the evenings. It turned out he only had anginal chest pain if he walked up a certain hill in the neighborhood after a full dinner, on a cool night, and after an argument with his wife. With any one of these, he could walk up the hill without angina. He got chest pain only if the full dinner, the argument with the wife, and cool weather were all present. That case has stuck in my mind. It illustrates the subtle combinations that sometimes can be teased out.

## 2.   *The patient has an identifiable psychosocial stress that produces the symptoms.*

Several patients in the book are good examples of people with symptoms produced by psychosocial stresses: In Chapter 11, you met Mrs. Carolyn Anderson, the divorcing mother with abdominal pains; Mr. Lonzo Craig, the truck driver with dizziness from a profane partner and a liberated wife; and Christine Swanson, who had diarrhea associated with an embezzling boss. In Chapter 8, there was Sweet Thing, with pains below her knees and with a false diagnosis of diabetes, tortured by the grief of her family. In Chapter 16, you met Joyce, with the recurring diabetic coma, who had to "show" her husband how much she needed attention.

## 3.   *The patient is unknowingly ingesting, inhaling, or coming into contact with a substance that is producing the symptoms.*

Patients in this category include Agnes, who had toothpaste diarrhea, and Dr. Jim, who absorbed his wife's vaginal estrogen cream and developed breast enlargement.

A colleague of mine, Dr. Allen Kaiser at Vanderbilt, told me of two patients where detective work led to identifying unusual offending substances. Both patients had recurring pneumonias. One of these turned out to be associated with the patient's sitting under an overhead insecticide spray when she worked at one particular desk at her husband's business. Most days she worked at other desks, avoiding the irritating spray. The other patient got pneumonia only when she helped her husband pack for his infrequent travels. They had put a powdered drying agent in the drawer with his clothes to prevent mildew, and when she removed the clothing, she inhaled the irritating particles that produced inflammation and pneumonia. Dr. Kaiser got to the root of these problems by persistently coaching the patients to explore their surroundings. The presence of medical diseases, particularly when they are recurring, should not preclude finding the offending agent. Obviously, medical care does not stop with a diagnosis.

### 4. The patient has a self-induced disease that produces the symptoms or findings.

Patients in this category can be most perplexing. In Chapter 19, you met Veronica, the nursing instructor who anticoagulated herself, produced bruises on her skin, falsified a fever, bled herself into anemia, and continued to bleed herself even while in the hospital.

Through the years, I have seen several patients with self-inflicted lesions and diseases. One woman feigned the pain of kidney stones and picked her gums with pecan shells to get some blood into her urine sample. Another patient regularly shook the thermometer upside down to produce false high-temperature readings. I had one patient when I was a resident who injected both insulin and heparin to produce a confounding combination of hypoglycemia and a bleeding disorder. Another patient injected bacteria under his skin to produce multiple abscesses. A beautiful young girl mutilated her legs with repeated injections of the insecticide Raid.

Sometimes the strange inflictions require partners. I have written of a young man who came into the hospital repeatedly with air under his skin (subcutaneous emphysema) and high fever (Meador 2003). No one could figure out this bizarre combination. He responded to antibiotics each time, only to return every few months. A sage member of the faculty finally got the real story. The young man and his girlfriend would meet late at night in the back of a store and have sexual intercourse. The girl, a bit kinky, liked to bite a small hole in the man's arm and pump him up with air from a bicycle pump. She liked the crunchy feel of the air under his skin. Sometimes he got infected and had to come into the hospital. One soon learns there are no bounds or limits to human behavior.

I was never able to follow any of these patients along. Except for Veronica, all left my practice as soon as I told them I knew what was going on. It is not within my apostolic function to be able to help these unfortunate people.

5. *The patient denies the existence or even the possibility of any biopsychosocial stress as a cause of the symptoms. Disease and symptoms have become a way of life. A subset of these patients is intent on defeating the physician by staying sick.*

This group of patients can be most trying. They are represented by all the patients in Group IV in Chapter 11. You will recall Mrs. Sarah Madison, the mother of three, with back pain and other symptoms, who denied any life stress in the face of two dysfunctional daughters. With her many symptoms, Florence in Chapter 10 initially fell into this group.

These patients are often difficult to interview and often change the subject quickly and adroitly. I once saw a patient who jumped from one symptom to another so quickly I could not follow her. I got the extreme idea of labeling several chairs in the exam room with body parts—one chair I labeled "stomach," another "chest," another "head," and still another "legs and feet." I looked at her with a perplexed feeling and said something like, "I am getting confused. You have so many problems, I cannot keep up." I enlisted her help. I asked that she move to the correct chair before launching into her symptoms in that area of the body. After she moved two or three times, she started laughing hysterically. It was funny, and I laughed along with her. Then she said, as Florence had finally said, "This is just ridiculous. Ridiculous." She continued laughing but also began to tell me a long and involved story of her unhappy marriage. I wish I had kept better notes on her case. She, like Florence, went on to a life free of symptoms and was able to accept help from a psychologist. I have no idea how the chairs worked, but they did.

These patients sometimes seem cut off from life. Disease and symptoms seem to be a way of life. You may remember Regina in Chapter 18, with whom I used the paradoxical approach of telling her she would never get well. She fit the pattern of one who likes to defeat experts. The only way she could defeat me was to get well—and she did, according to her husband, who called me from a phone booth. As I reflect on this whole group of patients, I think more and more of them fit the pattern of Regina. I only wish I had applied the paradox more often. I hope someone who reads these accounts will consider doing that and report the findings.

Some of these patients, like some patients with medical diseases, are using their symptoms to manipulate family members. All illness—even cancer—gives some gain to the patient. Sick people are granted all sorts of leeway and freedom that well people do not have. They are treated with kindness. Demands on them are reduced. Many people in this last category maintain their symptoms so they can remain in the sick role. Invalids are extreme examples of such people. I have found two telling questions that give clues to such behaviors.

First, "When were you last in excellent health?" The patients will say "never" or they cannot recall when they were ever in good health. One patient told me she had never been in good health since the obstetrician dropped her on the floor at her birth.

Second, "What would you do if all of your symptoms went away and you awoke one day in robust health?" The patient who is living with illness as a way of life will exhibit a look of puzzlement and confusion. Often he or she will have no answer.

•  •  •

As I look back over my long journey, I can still see Mrs. Gladys Goode paralyzed in her wheelchair in that old amphitheater. After the physostigmine injection, she stood and took a small bow, pointing us on our way to the seductive biomolecular model. Gradually, I came to a broader view of people and their diseases. My odyssey brought me to see that one is connected not only to organs and tissues but to spouses and families and culture and the whole biosphere.

Human communication is a large part of the broader model of treatment, yet scientific methods have still to observe and study much of human communication. It is time that we studied the doctor-patient relationship systematically and that we physicians found better ways to be in tune with the diverse human beings we see in our practices. If we are successful, there will be fewer patients who are labeled with diseases they do not have and more who have been guided toward healthier lives.

# Bibliography

Abram, Harry, and Clifton Meador. 1976. Introduction to *Basic Psychiatry for the Primary Care Physician*. Boston: Little, Brown.

Balint, Michael. 1955. "The Doctor, His Patient, and the Illness." *Lancet*, April 2, 683–88.

Bandler, Richard, and John Grinder. 1976a. *The Structure of Magic I*. Introduction by Virginia Satire and Gregory Bateson. Palo Alto: Science and Behavior Books.

_____. 1976b. *The Structure of Magic II*. Palo Alto: Science and Behavior Books.

_____. 1979. *Frogs into Princes*. Moab, Utah: Real People Press.

_____. 1982. *Reframing. Neurolinguistic Programming, and the Transformation of Meaning*. Moab, Utah: Real People Press.

Bateson, Gregory. 1982. *Steps to an Ecology of Mind: A Revolutionary Approach to Man's Understanding of Himself*. New York: Ballantine Books.

Bergman, A. B., and S. J. Stamm. 1967. "The Morbidity of Cardiac Nondisease in School Children." *NewEngland Journal of Medicine* 276:1008–13.

Cannon, Walter. 1957. "Voodoo Death." *Psychosomatic Medicine* 19:182–90. (Reprinted from *American Anthropologist* 44 [1942]).

Castelnuovo-Tedesco, Pietro. 1965. *The Twenty-Minute Hour: A Guide to Brief Psychotherapy for the Physician*. Boston: Little, Brown.

Dalai Lama and Daniel Goleman. 2003. *Destructive Emotions: A Scientific Dialogue with the Dalai Lama*. New York: Bantam Books.

Darwin, Charles. 1998. *The Expressions of the Emotions in Man and Animals*. 3d ed. New York: Oxford University Press.

DiRaimondo, Charles, Albert Roach, and Clifton Meador. 1980. "Gynecomastia, from Exposure to Vaginal Estrogen Cream." *New England Journal of Medicine* 302:1089–90.

Ekman, Paul. 2003. *Emotions Revealed.* New York: Times Books, Henry Holt.

Engel, George. 1977. "The Need for a New Medical Model: A Challenge for Biomedicine." *Science* 196:129–36.

Erickson, Milton, and Ernest Rossi. 1979. *Hypnotherapy: An Exploratory Casebook.* New York: Irvington.

Fleck, Ludwig. 1979. *Genesis and Development of a Scientific Fact.* Foreword by Thomas S. Kuhn. Chicago and London: University of Chicago Press.

Frank, Jerome, and Julia Frank. 1991. *Persuasion and Healing: A Comparative Study of Psychotherapy.* 3d ed. Baltimore and London: Johns Hopkins University Press.

Haley, Jay. 1986. *Uncommon Therapy: The Psychiatric Techniques of Milton Erickson, M.D.* New York: W.W. Norton.

———. 1987. *Transcript of Conversations with Milton H. Erickson, M.D.* On file at Milton Erickson Foundation. Phoenix: Triangle Press.

Harrison, Tinsley, ed. 1950. *Principles of Internal Medicine.* New York: Blakiston.

Hayakawa, S. I. 1978. *Language in Thought and Action.* 4th ed. San Francisco: Harcourt Brace Jovanovich.

Kuhn, Thomas. 1996. The Structure of Scientific Revolutions. 3d ed. Chicago and London: University of Chicago Press.

Lankton, Stephen, and Carol Lankton. 1983. *The Answer Within: A Clinical Framework of Ericksonian Hypnotherapy.* New York: Brunner/Mazel.

Meador, Clifton. 1965. "The Art and Science of Nondisease." *New England Journal of Medicine* 272:92–95.

———. 1991. "A Lament for Invalids." *Journal of the American Medical Association* 265:1374–75.

———. 1992a. "Hex Death: Voodoo Magic or Persuasion?" *Southern Medical Journal* 85:244–47.

———. 1992b. "Invalids: The Male Counterpart." *Southern Medical Journal* 85: 628–31.

———. 1992c. "The Person with the Disease." *Journal of the American Medical Association* 268:35.

———. 1992d. *A Little Book of Doctors' Rules.* Philadelphia: Hanley and Belfus.

_____. 1994. "The Last Well Person." *New England Journal of Medicine* 330:440.

_____. 2003. *Med School: A Collection of Stories, 1951 to 1955.* Nashville: Hillsboro Press.

Meador, Clifton, and Rosalie Lanius. 1995. "The Cryptic Error of Nondisease: The Hidden Power of Prevalence of Disease." *Journal of the Medical Association of Georgia* 84:316–22.

Odegaard, Charles. 1986. *Dear Doctor: A Personal Letter to a Physician.* Menlo Park, Calif.: Henry J. Kaiser Family Foundation.

Roeuché, Berton. 1947. *Eleven Blue Men.* Boston: Little, Brown.

_____. 1988. *The Medical Detectives.* New York: Truman Talley Books.

_____. 1995. *The Man Who Grew Two Breasts.* New York: Truman Talley Books/Dutton.

Rogers, Carl. 1961. *On Becoming a Person.* 2d ed. Boston: Houghton Mifflin.

Sapira, Joseph. 1999. *The Art and Science of Bedside Diagnosis.* Baltimore: Williams and Wilkins.

Soden, Kevin. 2003. *The Art of Medicine.* Philadelphia: Mosby.

St. Clair, Carmen, and John Grinder. 2001. *Whispering in the Wind.* Scotts Valley, Calif.: J. and C. Enterprises.

Walker, Lewis. 2002. *Consulting with NLP: Neurolinguistic Programming in the Medical Consultation.* Abingdon, U.K.: Radcliffe Medical Press.

Watzlawick, P., J. Weakland, and R. Fisch. 1974. *Change.* New York: Norton.

Wennberg, J. E., and A. Gittelsohn. 1982. "Variations in Medical Care among Small Areas." *New England Journal of Medicine* 314:512–14.

Zeig, Jeffrey. 1982. *Ericksonian Approaches to Hypnosis and Psychotherapy.* New York: Brunner/Mazel.

# Index

Abram, Harry S., xi, xiii–xiv, 63–64, 150–52
abscess, 152, 160
acromegaly, 91
Adelaine, 114–23
adrenal glands, 45–46, 109
adrenal hyperplasia, 45, 47
Agnes, 102–6, 159
allergies, 75
Amy, 9–14, 126
Anderson, Carolyn, 84–85, 159
anemia, 33, 158, 160
angina pectoris, 158–59
antibiotics, 160
anticoagulant, 151
antidepressants, 71
APCs, 143
apomorphine, 29
apostolic function, x–xi, 100, 154, 161
appendectomy, 41–42
appendicitis, 40
Art and Science of Bedside Diagnosis, The, 51
"Art and Science of Nondisease," xii

arthritis, 34
aspirin, 143
atrophic vaginitis, 111–12
atrophy (muscles), 139
attentive rapport, 99

Bachelor Officer's Quarters (BOQ), 8
back pain, 87–88, 142–49, 161
Balint, Michael, x–xi, xiv, 100, 154
Bandler, Richard, 99, 118–19, 127
barium enema, 86
Barrymore, Lionel, 25
Basic Psychiatry for the Primary Care Physician, xi
BBC television, 31
Bellevue Hospital, 6
bicycle pump, 161
biochemical rib, 48
biomolecular model
  and cognitive dissonance, 19
  and diabetes, 9
  and false diagnosis, xii–xiii
  and hex death, 32
  hypothetical statement, xi

biomolecular model *(continued)*
    and Clifton Meador, 4
    as research tool, x
    and the scientific method,
        22–23
    and Sweet Thing, 59–60
    and U.S. medicine, ix
biopsychosocial model of disease,
    xiii–xiv, 50, 155
bladder infection, 144
bladder-neck obstruction, 68, 70,
    75
blood-loss anemia, 153
brine test, 18
bronchitis, 75
bruises, 150–54, 160
burning lips, 143

caffeine, 143
calomel, 23
cancer, 43, 109
Cannon, Walter, 31–32
carbonic acid, 124
Center for the Study of the Person,
    xiv, 53
cerebral aneurysm, 91
chairs, as body part analogy,
    161–62
*Change*, 144
client-centered therapy, 52
clinicopathological conferences
    (CPC), 67
codeine, 143
cognitive dissonance, 19
colitis, 75
colon, 34, 75, 103, 107
Columbia Presbyterian Hospital,
    5–6, 10

communication, auditory/visual,
    130–32, 157, 163
congenital adrenal hyperplasia,
    45, 47
Conley, Joseph, 97–98
Conley, Susan, 97–98
Conrad, Frances. *See* Miss Cootsie
constipation, 143
contentless inquiry, 104
conversion symptoms, 39,
    133–34
cortisone, 144
coumadin, 91
Craig, Lonzo, 85–86, 159
Crest toothpaste, 106, 159
"crock," xiv, 61
Crohn's disease, 86
"Cryptic Error of Nondisease: The
    Hidden Power of Prevalence of
    Disease, The," 93–94
cuing, 100–101
Cushing syndrome, 81, 158

D&C, 144
dead-end diagnoses, 103
Demerol, 143
Department of Family Medicine,
    University of South Alabama
    School of Medicine, 96
depression
    and Adelaine, 114
    excluded from patient group
        analysis, 82
    and Florence's symptoms, 80
    and hospitals, 126
    treatment for, 39
desiccant, 159–60
diabetes mellitus. *See also* type 1
    diabetes

and Adelaine, 114
and the biomolecular model, 9
Sweet Thing, 55–56, 91, 159
diabetic ketoacidosis, 10, 124–25,
    132, 159
diarrhea, 102–6, 159
Dilaudid, 143
Discovery Health Channel, 31
disseminated histoplasmosis, 135
diverticulosis, 103
Doane's back-pain pills, 143
Doherty, Drayton
    develops pneumonia, 33
    and false diagnosis, 75
    and Johnson, Irene, 20
    medical training, 23
    and Miss Cootsie, 23–24, 26
    and Vance Vanders, 27–31, 79
Dr. Jim, 108–13
dropped kidneys, 34, 75

ecchymoses, 150
electromyograms, 135
electroshock therapy, 114
Eleven Blue Men, 113
emotional states, 127–28
emphysema, 34, 160–61
endocrinology, 35–36
enema, barium, 86
Engel, George, xiii, 50–51, 155
Erickson, Milton, 99, 157
estrogen, 48, 109, 110–12
Eugene, 40–47

factitial diseases, 151–54, 161
fainting, 18–19
Fairhope, Alabama, xiv, 95–101,
    155
fallopian tubes, 41

false diagnosis
    and the biomolecular model,
        xii–xiii
    and Florence's symptoms, 75
    studies on, 93–94
    in SUO groups, 90–93
    and Sweet Thing, 56–57, 159
    table, 93
family medicine, 96
fever of unknown origin (FUO),
    xiv
fibrosis, 44
Florence, 66–74, 88, 91, 161
Floyd, 143, 147–49
Foley catheter, 124
Fort Hood, Texas, 5–9, 17–18
Fourth Armored Division, 6, 7
Frank, Jerome, 100
full rapport, 138, 155–56

gallbladder disease, 86
gallstones, 81
gastritis, 75
gastroenteritis, 75
gastrointestinal malabsorption,
    86, 158
genetic transmission, 32
genome, x, 32
Gladys, 111–12
glucocorticoids, 91
glucose, 91
glucose tolerance test, 57, 58
God, 138, 141
goiter, 24–26, 81
gonorrhea, 7
Goode, Gladys, 1–3, 163
grant funding, 101
Grinder, John, 99, 118–19, 127
gynecomastia, 108, 110

Harrison, Tinsley, 158
Harrison's Principles of Internal
    Medicine, 158
Harvard, 31
headaches, 114–23, 143
Headquarters, Headquarters
    Company, 7–8
heart disease, 93
heat exhaustion, 16
heat stroke, 15–19
hematocrit, 153
hemorrhoids, 81
heparin, 151, 152
hernia, 34, 75
herniated disc, 88
hex death, 31–32
"Hex Death: Voodoo Magic or
    Persuasion," 31–32
hiatus hernia, 34, 75
house calls, 24
Human Dimensions in Medicine,
    52–53
hypercalcemia, 158
hypertension, 81
hyperthyroid, 25
hyperthyroidism, 81, 91, 158
hypochondriasis, 39
hypoglycemia, 85, 138, 160
hypoglycemic reactions, 56
hyponatremia, 158
hypopituitarism, 81, 158
hypopotassemia, 158
hypothyroidism, 21–22, 22, 158
hysterectomy, 41, 45, 87–88, 90
hysteria, 39
hysterical (conversion symptoms),
    133–34
hysterical paralysis, 137

impending detached retina, 68
incongruence, 128–29
infectious mononucleosis, 134–35
insecticide spray, 159
insulin, 9, 11, 55, 124. *See also*
    Amy; Sweet Thing
*International Classification of
    Diseases*, 82
invalids, 24, 26, 162
irritable bowel, 103, 107
itching legs, 143

Johns Hopkins School of Medicine,
    52
Johnson, Irene, 20–22, 26, 158
Joyce, 124–32, 159
juvenile-onset diabetes mellitus,
    9–14

Kaiser, Allen, 159–60
kidney infection, 80
kidney stones, 160
kidneys, 34, 75
Killeen, Texas, 6
kinesthetic systems, 157
King, William, 1–2
Kirkpatrick, Sam, Sr., 30
kitten, 13, 126
Korean War, 5, 15, 158
Kuhn, Thomas, xiii
Kussmaul breathing, 124

*la belle indifférence*, 133
La Jolla, California, xiv
leg pain, 55–56
legs, itching, 143
Lente, 11
lice, 78–79
Liddle, Grant, 54

lipoma, 91
Little Cootsie, 24
lizard, 29
Loeb, Robert F., 10
low blood sugar, 34
lung cancer, 109
lymphoma, 91

Madison, Sarah, 87–88, 161
malignant lymphoma, 91
malingering, 137
Man Who Grew Two Breasts, The, 113
Marie, 133–41
masculinizing/androgen-secreting tumor, 46
McGregor, Red, 15–19
Meador, Clifton K.
    and Berton Roueché, 113
    and Carl Rogers, 52–53, 157
    Columbia Presbyterian Hospital residency, 5–6
    dean, School of Medicine at University of Alabama, 49
    faculty at University of Alabama, 35–37
    at Fairhope, Alabama, 95–101
    and Harry S. Abram, 63–64
    "Hex Death: Voodoo Magic or Persuasion," 31–32
    interviewing techniques, 155–56
    military service. See Fort Hood, Texas
    on the mind/body dichotomy, 37–39
    and physician-directed recollection (PDR), xv, 156–57

Saint Thomas Hospital in Nashville, 54, 102
    and self-inflected disease, 154
    Selma practice, xii, 20–22
    specialist in sexual differentiation disorders, 40
medical care, dissatisfaction with, xii
Medical Detectives, 113
medical diagnosis, 33–34, 36
medical slang (derogatory), xiv, 61
migraine headache, 75
mind/body dichotomy, 37–39, 50
miscarriage, 143–44
Miss Cootsie, 23–26
Mobile, Alabama, xiv, 95
molecular genetics, x
morphine, 143
Mullins, H.C. "Moon," xiv, 96–97
myasthenia gravis, 1–3, 9
myelograms, 135, 142
myositis, 135

nausea, 143
"Need for a New Medical Model: A Challenge for Biomedicine, The," 50–51
New England Journal of Medicine, xii, 113
New Yorker, 113
N.I.H. Clinical Research Center, 35
nocebo effect, 32
NPH insulin, 11, 55
Nuclear Medicine Laboratory, 33

On Becoming a Person, 53
ovaries, 41, 44, 46
overlapping, 119

paralysis, 133–41
paralysis (hysterical), 133–34, 137
paranoid schizophrenic, 69
Pavlovian response, 121, 122
penicillin, 26
peripheral neuropathy, 56
pernicious anemia, 33
phenacetin, 143
phlebitis, 91
physician-directed recollection
    (PDR), xv, 156–57
*Physicians' Desk Reference*, xv
physostigmine, 3, 163
placebo effect
    and Amy, 14
    and Florence's symptoms, 80
    and hex death, 32
    and medical diagnosis, 33–34,
        36
"Placebo" television show, 31
pneumonia, 26, 33, 159–60
Point Clear, 96
porphyria cutanea tarda, 81
porphyrias, 158
prednisone, 11–12
propylthiouracil, 91
protamine sulfate, 151
protamine zinc insulin, 11
protein-bound iodine level, 21
proteomics, x, 32
psychiatry, 38–39

Qwell lotion, 79

radioiodine uptake, 21
Regina, 142–49, 162
renal glycosuria, 57, 58
retina, 68

retroverted/tilted uterus, 34
rheumatoid arthritis, 34
ringing ears, 143
Riven, Sam, 1–3
Robert Wood Johnson Foundation,
    The, 52
Rogerian psychotherapy, 52
Rogers, Carl
    and Florence's symptoms, 67–
        68, 71, 73
    and Clifton Meador, xiv, 52–
        53, 155, 157
Rogers, David, 52
Roueché, Berton, 113

Saint Thomas Hospital in
    Nashville, 54
salt tablets, 16
Sapira, Joseph, xiv, 50, 51, 155
Schilling test, 33
scientific method, 22–23
Scott White Clinic, 12
Selma, Alabama, xii, 33
semi Lente, 11
sensitivity sessions, 53
"shad," xiv, 61
sinus, 75
skin rashes, 143
somatizing disorder, 82
somatoform disorder, 39
spastic colon, 34, 75, 103, 107
sperm count, 43
spinal tap, 114, 135
Stickney, Stonewall, xiv, 97–100
stroke, 91
strychnine, 23
subcutaneous emphysema, 160–61
Swanson, Christine, 86–87, 159

Sweet Thing
  diabetes and leg pain, 55–60
  false diagnosis, 91, 159
  as Group IV patient, 88
  and Marie, 138
sympathetic illness, examples, 19
symptoms of unknown origin
  (SUO)
  categories for, 64–65, 157–62
  clinical approach, 61–63
  defined, xiv–xv
  Florence's list, 71–72
  patient group analysis, 81–84
  patient groups defined, **89**
  and psychiatry, 39
  and Veronica, 150–54
syphilis, 7

T groups, 53–54
tachycardia, 85
Temple, Texas, 6
testicles, 42–43
testicular cancer, 43, 109
testosterone, 48
*Textbook of Medicine*, 10
therapeutic paradox, 144–45, 146,
  162
thyroid extract, 25
thyroid gland, 22
thyroiditis, 91
thyroxine, 22

tri-iodothyronine, 22
true hermaphrodites, 41, 46
"turkey," xiv, 61
type 1 diabetes, 9–14

ulcerative colitis, 86
undescended testicles, 42–43, 45
United Kingdom, x
University of Alabama, xiv, 158
University of Alabama School of
  Medicine, 35–37
University of South Alabama
  School of Medicine, xiv
uterus, 34, 41, 45

vaginitis, 111–12
Vanderbilt University, 54
Vanders, Vance, 27–31
varicose veins, 81
Veronica, 150–54, 160
virilizing adrenal hyperplasia, 45
vitamin deficiencies, 158
vitamins, 110–11
voodoo, 28, 30

Walter Reed Hospital, 11
watering eyes, 143
weak kidneys, 34
witch doctor, 28
worm infestations, 158